For the people

'May all beings have happiness and the causes of happiness.

May all beings be free from suffering and the causes of suffering.

May all beings never be parted from freedom's true joy.

May all beings dwell in equanimity, free from attachment and aversion'.

Buddhist Prayer

YOU ARE THE CURE

ALCHEMICAL
EDITION

CHRIS JUSTES

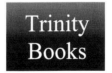

United Kingdom
www.trinitybooks.co.uk

Published by Trinity Books,
United Kingdom.
www.trinitybooks.co.uk

The information within this book is for
educational purposes only and is not intended as a
substitute for the medical advice of physicians. The
reader should regularly consult a physician in
matters relating to his/her health and particularly
with respect to any symptoms that may require
diagnosis or medical attention.

YOU ARE THE CURE

It was after years of suffering from depression and addiction that I finally discovered *'The Cure'*. I tried a number of treatments out in the past with some success, but nothing came close to *The Cure*.

The Cure is a simple solution to addiction that can also alleviate many other illnesses that are related to neurochemical imbalances within the body and can be triggered using everyday products that you can buy in a grocery store for next to nothing.

There are a number of treatments available for neurochemical disorders such as depression and addiction, but I have found that *The Cure* is the quickest and easiest way to reset the chemistry of the body and end the cycle of addiction.

My journey began years ago as a teenager when I was addicted to alcohol, nicotine and junk food. As a drinker I got into a lot of trouble and despite the negative consequences alcohol had on my life I still drank to fit in as alcohol gave me a confidence boost and helped me lose my inhibitions.

Alcohol got rid of my anxiety but later on in life it became an issue as I used alcohol to alleviate my depression and any negative thoughts and feelings that I had about myself and my life. Once the binge drinking was over, however, the depression and anxiety were still there as alcohol was only a temporary solution to my problems and made matters worse.

Alcoholism runs in my family and I had lost a family member through alcoholism and depression. It was a difficult time for me and my family to deal with during my drinking years, but I would not change it for the world because without my struggle I would not have discovered *The Cure.*

The turning point of my life began in 2008 when I decided to face my inner demons after running away from them for so many years. I always thought in the back of my mind that if I had a loving family, a good job and stayed away from alcohol and negative people that my life would get better. Life gave me all of this but still, the pain remained, so I had no choice but to face the pain head on and it was best decision I ever made.

Facing my inner demons was the catalyst for my spiritual awakening which led me on an inward journey of self-discovery, self-love and eventually to *The Cure*.

For the past 10 years, I have been free from binge drinking, nicotine addiction and depression and after reading this book and trying *The Cure* out for yourself, you can be free from addiction (and possibly other illnesses) too.

Contents

References

What is Addiction?

An addiction is a neurochemical dependency on a substance, place, object or activity that makes you feel good, and a sense of worth derives from it.

Addictions are often characterised by the inability to stop the activities we are addicted to despite the negative consequences they may have on our health and wellbeing. Some addicts, however, do not have the desire to stop their harmful habits as they do not see their addictions as a problem as the effects of their addictions are manageable, denied and/or socially accepted.

We become addicted to the feelings derived from our actions and not the things themselves unless the things themselves mimic our internal chemistry as in the case of drugs, alcohol and junk food. If no pleasure or comfort derived from the things that we were addicted to, we would not have been addicted to them.

Addictions are chemical-based and have an effect on our neurochemistry. The feel-good chemicals of the brain - gamma-aminobutyric acid (GABA), serotonin, dopamine, endorphins and oxytocin quell the negative thoughts, feelings and emotions that we have on a daily basis. When we are low in these feel-good chemicals, we begin to feel unpleasant and crave that which makes us feel good and we self-medicate in an attempt to readdress the neurochemical imbalance within and return to homeostasis (a state of rest/ internal balance).

Cravings and withdrawal symptoms are the body's way of telling us that we are low in the neurochemicals that are needed to feel-good and function normally as the body cannot function properly without a certain number of neurochemicals that are needed to carry out its daily functions.

The feel-good chemicals of the brain also regulate the physical functions of the body such as the modulation of pain, sleeping patterns and temperature control. Withdrawal symptoms such as hot flushes, restless-ness, discomfort and pain are due to the lack of feel-good chemicals within which cause us to feel unpleasant - mentally, physically and emotionally.

The withdrawal symptoms that we experience when we are low in the feel-good chemicals are one of the main reasons why we reach for the things that give us pleasure and ease the discomfort of withdrawing from that which we are lacking internally.

When we have substances that mimic our internal chemistry, our cells react and are programmed to alter their chemical set points (from a homeostatic set point to an allostatic set point) to adapt to the external source of feel-good chemicals. As a direct result of this, we become dependent on the external source of feel-good chemicals because we have programmed our cells to want more feel-good chemicals than usual. Overstimulation from supernormal stimuli such as drugs, alcohol, junk food or trauma program our cells to want more of the feel-good chemicals than is normally required.

Some of the treatments that are available for depression and addiction restore the feel-good chemicals of the brain to functional levels. Antidepressant medications such as Selective Serotonin Reuptake Inhibitors (SSRI's) target the serotonin synapses (connections between nerve cells) in the brain and increase serotonin levels.

SSRIs alter the genes of cells changing their chemical set points. Anti-addiction medications work in a similar way and bind to specific receptors of the brain, reducing cravings and withdrawal symptoms to the point of not wanting the things we were addicted to. Anti-addiction medications reprogram our cells, so we no longer depend on an external source of feel-good chemicals to feel good by changing our chemical set

3

points to what they should be (from allostatic to homeostatic).

Most of the antidepressant and anti-addiction medications (with the exception of some entheogens & entactogens) require a prolonged course of medication to be effective and are known to have side effects that can be harmful to our health and wellbeing. There is, however, an easier way to reprogram our cells and change the chemistry of the brain (and gut flora) that only takes one hour or so to do and has minimal side effects that are harmful to our health when done correctly. I have found that the quickest and easiest way to end the cycle of addiction/craving is to enter into ketosis, *The Cure* that exists within all of us.

Ketosis

Ketosis has been used as a medical intervention for over 2000 years to treat a number of physical and neurological disorders. Scientific evidence and anecdotal reports suggest that ketosis and a ketogenic diet can be used to treat a wide range of conditions such as epilepsy, diabetes, obesity, depression, addiction, schizophrenia and even some types of cancer.

Ketosis is a natural physiological metabolic state where the body uses ketones (ketone bodies) as its main source of fuel instead of glucose. Ketone bodies are water-soluble lipid molecules that are produced in the liver by ketogenesis and the two main ketone bodies used for fuel when we are in ketosis are 3-beta-hydroxybutyrate and acetoacetate.

Ketogenesis occurs when carbohydrate levels are low, and/or when caffeine levels are high and/or when there is an increase in fatty acids or ketones in the bloodstream. When either of these conditions are met the body begins to breakdown fats via ketogenesis converting them into ketone bodies from Acetyl Coenzyme A (Acetyl-CoA).

The ketone bodies are converted back into Acetyl-CoA via the Krebs cycle (also known as the Citric acid or Tricarboxylic acid cycle) and then made into an available source of chemical energy called Adenosine triphosphate (ATP). The ATP produced in the mitochondria of the liver becomes the available source of energy for the brain, organs, muscles and cells and is the precursor to DNA and RNA.

I have found that ketosis can be induced in a number of ways through water fasting, dry fasting, a low carbohydrate diet, tea, coffee, cacao, coconut, ketones, caffeine and some adaptogens such as Rhodiola and St John's Wort.

Ketosis is typically induced through fasting or dietary changes such as switching to a low carbohydrate diet, but with these methods, it usually takes around 48 hours for women and 72 hours for men to enter ketosis.

With the typical methods of entering ketosis, we go through carbohydrate or drug withdrawals until we enter ketosis and this can be difficult to deal with. Withdrawal symptoms usually include cravings (for drugs or foods high in carbohydrates), obsessive thoughts (about the food or substances we are addicted to), headaches, cramps, muscle weakness, light-headedness, stress, discomfort, pain, disturbed sleeping patterns and extreme hunger.

Tea, coffee, cacao, coconut and caffeine, on the other hand, can induce ketosis within hours and skip the process of carbohydrate or drug withdrawals. We can enter ketosis within 1 hour by consuming coconut or caffeine containing substances such as cacao, tea, coffee or caffeine tablets. I have induced ketosis within hours to break the cycle of addiction, treat depression, correct gut flora imbalances, improve my eyesight and stabilise my blood sugar levels.

From a chemical point of view, ketosis can correct a number of neurochemical and hormonal imbalances that manifest as diseases. The neuro-correcting aspect of ketosis may be due to the increased activity of gamma-aminobutyric acid (GABA), the brain's main inhibitory neurotransmitter.

Increases in GABA levels decrease glutamate activity in the brain. Glutamate is the brain's main excitatory neurotransmitter which accounts for more than 90% of the brain's synaptic connections. Glutamate is also the precursor of GABA and the most prevalent neuro-transmitter in the brain.

Some neuroscientists speculate that glutamate imbalances within the brain are responsible for the cycles of addiction and that addictions are the result of the brain trying to maintain glutamate homeostasis.

Trauma also causes glutamate overstimulation in the brain which may explain why trauma is a gateway drug for some that often leads to addiction.

Researchers have found that all addictions activate the dopamine reward pathways of the brain whether the addictions are to heroin, cocaine, pornography, sex, gambling, nicotine, alcohol or sugar. All addictive substances and hedonistic behaviours activate the dopamine reward pathways of the brain that are regulated by glutamate-containing neurons.

Glutamate has been hypothesised to be involved in other illnesses that are related to neurochemical imbalances within the brain such as posttraumatic stress disorder (PTSD), epilepsy, depression, obsessive-compulsive disorder (OCD), dementia, schizophrenia and autism which may explain why ketosis works for a wide range of mental illnesses by correcting the GABA/glutamate ratios in the brain.

What Ketosis and a Ketogenic diet can treat, prevent or improve.

Scientific evidence	Anecdotal reports
Acne	
Addiction	Addiction
Adenylosuccinate lyase deficiency	
Ageing	
Alzheimer disease	
Amyotrophic lateral sclerosis	
Angelman syndrome	
Anxiety	Anxiety
Appetite disorders: -	Appetite disorders: -
Anorexia, Binge eating,	Anorexia, Binge eating, Bulimia,
Food addiction	Food addiction
Attention deficit hyperactivity disorder	
Autism	
Bipolar disorder	Bipolar disorder
Blood pressure	Blood pressure

Brain Trauma	
	Breathing problems
Cancer: - Astrocytoma, Breast, Colon, Glioblastoma, Head, Liver, Lung, Malignant brain, Malignant glioma, Neck, Neuroblastoma, Pancreatic, Prostate, Squamous cell carcinoma (SCC), Stomach cancer	
Cardiac ischemia	
CDKL5 encephalopathy	
Cognitive impairment	
Cortical malformations	
Craving	
Crohn's disease	

Depression	
Diabetes	
Dementia	
Doose syndrome	
Dravet syndrome	
Endurance	Endurance
Energy levels	
Epilepsy	
Fertility	
Glaucoma	
GLUT-1 deficiency	
Gut flora	
Heart disease	
HIV-associated neurocognitive disorders	
Hormonal imbalances	Hormonal imbalances
Huntington's disease	Huntington's disease
Increases VO2 ratio	Increases VO2 ratio
Infantile spasms	Infantile spasms
Inflammation	Inflammation
Irritable bowel syndrome	Irritable bowel syndrome
Lafora body disease	
Landau-Kleffner syndrome	

Lennox-Gastaut syndrome	
McArdle disease	
Mitochondrial disorders	
Mood disorder	Mood
Multiple Sclerosis	
Narcolepsy	
Nonalcoholic fatty liver disease	
Neuroprotective	
Obesity	Obesity
Ohtahara syndrome	
Pain reduction	Pain reduction
Parkinson's disease	
Phosphofructokinase deficiency	
Polycystic ovary syndrome	
	Posttraumatic stress disorder
Pyruvate dehydrogenase deficiency	
Protects/repairs DNA	
Rett syndrome	
Rheumatoid arthritis	

Schizophrenia	Schizophrenia
Seizures	
Sex life	
Sleep disturbances	
	Stabilizes blood sugar levels
Stress	
Stroke	
Subacute Sclerosing panencephalitis	
Tuberous sclerosis complex	
	Ulcerative colitis
Weight loss	Weight loss
Well-being	Well-being
Withdrawals	Withdrawals

Coconut Ketosis

Please read all of the instructions before you begin.

What to do:

- Take 25g (around 5 heaped medium sized tea-spoons) of raw (cold-pressed) virgin coconut oil in one go and drink it down with a cup or 8oz glass of water.

  Wait around 20 to 45 minutes to enter ketosis and drink nothing but water (spring or distill-ed) during and after the process for at least 1 hour after you have entered ketosis.

Before you begin:

- Wait at least 30 to 60 minutes after a meal or drink (with the exception of water) before trying coconut ketosis as food in the colon can interfere with the process. Coconut ketosis works well first thing in the morning on an empty stomach.

- You can mix other ingredients with the coconut oil (to make coconut ice cream etc.) to make it taste better as long as there is at least 25g of coconut oil for it to work and no more than 60 - 80g of sugar in total but this may differ for each of us.

  Store-bought coconut ice cream with a high coconut oil content works that contains other ingredients such as unrefined sugar and flavourings. Fresh or desiccated coconut meat (around 50g) works too if you are not a fan of coconut oil.

  Adding half a teaspoon of cayenne and black pepper to coconut oil or coconut meat will get you into ketosis off half the recommended dose (13g oil/25g meat) as cayenne and black pepper increase the bioavailability, absorption and metabolism of medium chain triglycerides (MCT's) found in coconut oil that triggers ketosis.

  If you are not a fan of cayenne pepper, just use black pepper as it is the black pepper that allows you to have half the recommended dose to enter ketosis. Be sure to reduce the sugar content respectively if spices are used in the recipe to 30 - 40g of sugar in total including the sugars naturally found in food.

If you have never tried coconut ketosis before I do not recommend mixing the coconut oil with other ingredients initially, so you get an idea of what coconut ketosis is about.

- Do alone as the energy of others (including pets) can affect the process unless the others involved are not giving out negative energy or conditioning you and the process with their opinions or desires (subconscious or other-wise).

  If you live on a busy street, it may be a good idea to close the curtains or blinds to avoid others conditioning you. Emotions and thoughts are electrical in nature and have an effect on our neurochemistry. Avoid social media sites or contact with people via touch or technology and do not hold or wear any crystals/gems/metal jewellery or use a grounding mat or sheet as they can interfere with the process.

- If you have any medical conditions or are taking any medication, try coconut ketosis supervised initially to avoid any complications.

What to expect:

- Mental calm.
- No mental highs or lows.
- No blood sugar highs or lows.
- Improved eyesight.
- Increased mental concentration.
- Increased mental and physical energy.
- A balanced mind.
- Diminished appetite.
- An increase in breathing and a need for more air.
- No withdrawals or cravings for the things you were addicted to.

Typical symptoms of ketosis:
(include but not always).

- Cold shins and hands.
- Increased mental alertness.
- Increased concentration and focus.
- Tense shoulders.
- Feeling limber/supple joints.
- Increased strength in the legs and spinal column.
- Occasional mental calmness.
- Tears (for first timers only but not always).
- An increase in confidence.
- Feeling thirsty.

- Slight nausea.
- Bad breath (ketone breath).
- Tongue sticking to the roof of your mouth.
- Feeling angry/stressed/emotional (due to the release of toxins).
- Increased sense of smell.
- Horrible taste in your mouth from ketones.
- Stomach-ache (coconut oil draws toxins from your stomach/intestines).
- Runny nose (keto flu).

What to consider:

- If this is your first-time entering ketosis and you have lived a very toxic lifestyle, when you enter ketosis, you may cry as toxins are released into the bloodstream. Tears are one way the body releases toxins. This is fine and nothing to worry about as entering ketosis breaks down body fat where toxins are stored.

- Have plenty of sodium, around 4000 - 7000mg (about 2 - 3 teaspoons/15 - 18g of salt) the day before and/or on the day. Ketosis releases sodium from the kidneys as it lowers insulin levels in the body, the hormone that regulates blood sugar levels and appetite.

If you eat a standard western diet sodium is not something to worry about, but if you eat a low sodium diet, a little extra sodium will help. The body's sodium requirements increase when you follow a ketogenic diet or enter ketosis regularly.

Sometimes it is common to crave salty junk food after entering ketosis, but it is the sodium the body craves that is in the junk food and not the junk food per se. If you crave salty food after you have entered ketosis then you have not had enough sodium prior to entering ketosis. Eat something high in sodium to satisfy the cravings for salty food.

Good sources of sodium:

— Sea salt (2338mg per 6g).
— Himalayan salt (1080mg per 6g).
— Sea vegetables - Seaweed, Algae (Kombu highest @ 2727mg per 100g).
— Samphire (2500mg per 100g).
— Beet greens (226mg per 100g).
— Swiss chard (213mg per 100g).
— Celery (80mg per 100g).

• If you have anything that once caused an addiction after entering ketosis, it will restart the cycle of addiction again to the substance that you were addicted to by altering the chemistry of the brain and disrupting homeostasis. You will need to enter ketosis again to stop the cycle of addiction and reset the chemistry of the brain/gut flora.

We become addicted to things because those substances whether they are food or drugs alter our neurochemistry and as a result, our bodies crave such substances to readdress the chemical imbalance within and return to homeostasis. We can however, control our substance/food use while in ketosis for example if we had an addiction to alcohol/junk food where we binged to the point of excess (when out of ketosis), while in ketosis we can have one beer or packet of crisps and leave it at that, but if we get out of ketosis by going over the carbohydrate threshold (beer and crisps both being carbohydrates) it will start the binge cycle of addiction again and cravings will compel us to have more beer or crisps until we enter ketosis again to stop the cycle of addiction/cravings.

I have found that bingeing only happens again when we have not been abstinent for a long period of time as our brains and neural networks are still wired/programmed to binge. If we have been abstinent for years and are familiar with entering ketosis, the neural networks that supported our binge patterns of behaviour will no longer exist as our tolerance to substances is a direct result of how many neural networks we have built up over the years.

Ketosis allows us to have the substances we were once addicted to in a controlled manner if we remain in ketosis or re-enter ketosis. Ketosis gives us the freedom to choose when and what to consume in a way that suits us as ketosis gives us the freedom over food and substances when our nutritional needs are met. Some people only eat one meal a day (OMAD diet) as opposed to three main meals a day, and some people eat even less than that thanks to the power of ketosis (Inedia/ Breatharians).

Once you have entered ketosis, you do not need to stay in ketosis for more than an hour for it to reset the chemistry of the brain/gut flora. After that it is up to you what to do. You can stay in ketosis if you like or get yourself out of ketosis by eating around 90 grams or more of carbohydrates in one sitting.

If you want to remain in ketosis keep your carbohydrate intake low (around 20 - 70g per day not including fibre). If you want to get in and out of ketosis throughout the day for whatever reason, the amount of carbohydrates you have throughout the day is irrelevant when you enter ketosis using coconuts (unless you have an unusually high amount of carbohydrates throughout the day).

- Dose may vary depending on the quality of the coconut used, whether the coconut is raw or has been cooked, your digestion, your body weight and what the coconut has been mixed with.

  If coconut ketosis does not work the first-time experiment with a larger or smaller dose and/or add cayenne and black pepper the next time and see what works best for you, or altern-atively use a different method to enter ketosis.

Additional information:

- For best results enter ketosis nutritionally and make sure you have eaten well the day before and/or on the day to feel the full benefits of entering ketosis. Have plenty of citrus fruit as the citric acid in the fruit helps with the Krebs/ Citric acid cycle and energy levels.

  Once ketosis sets in you should feel great and full of vigour. If you feel weak or low, it is because you have not addressed a nutritional deficiency that existed prior to entering ketosis.

Ketosis will still work and reset the chemical set points of the body but should be followed up by meeting the body's nutritional needs i.e., a plant-based whole food alkaline diet.

- Fresh coconut meat, coconut milk or coconut butter is best, followed by raw coconut oil, but cooked or dried coconut can be used too depending on your preference as long as there is around 25g of coconut oil in the coconut product to trigger ketosis.

  Raw coconut cleanses the liver and colon due to its high vibrational energy and nutritional content. Fresh coconuts are minimally processed and contain live enzymes which ease the body's role of digesting and assimilating the nutrients we get from food.

- Too much coconut oil has a laxative effect. Your body will naturally tell you when you have had enough coconut oil (this is usually around 30 - 50g in one go).

- Entering ketosis uses up reserves of sodium and vitamin B12 so be sure to have plenty if you enter ketosis on a regular basis. Be sure to have at least 4000 - 7000mg of sodium per day (about 2 - 3 teaspoons/15 - 18g of salt).

The Hydroxocobalamin or Methylcobalamin forms of vitamin B12 are the best bioavailable forms of B12 to use as they have the highest absorption rate. I recommend taking a high strength Methylcobalamin (vitamin B12) sublingual supplement of 1000mcg or more (daily) if you enter ketosis on a regular basis.

If you get pins and needles (a numbing of the fingers and toes) after entering ketosis it is a sign of vitamin B12 deficiency, so be sure to get your vitamin B12 levels checked at the doctors and supplement immediately.

Use a good quality sea salt or rock salt such as Himalayan salt or a natural unrefined sea salt (free from anti-caking agents). Table salt has been linked to health problems such as high blood pressure, kidney disease and an increased risk of heart attacks.

- Do not use tap water as tap water contains pollutants and contaminants that are harmful to our health. Tap water contains endocrine disruptors, hormones, plastics, pesticides, heavy metals, medications, nitrates and fertilisers.

The pollutants found in tap water have been found to cause neurological disorders and have been linked to hormonal disruptions, cancer and Alzheimer's disease. Use a good quality water such as spring or distilled water that does not contain the harmful impurities found in tap water.

- The best way to tell if you have entered ketosis is to see if your tongue is sticking to the roof of your mouth and you have an increased need for air. You may also notice an improvement in concentration, focus, eyesight and sense of smell.

  If you are unsure whether you have entered ketosis buy some ketone test strips and test your urine for ketones 2 - 6 hours after entering ketosis or first thing in the morning the following day.

  After following a ketogenic diet for a while and/or entering ketosis regularly, the ketone test strips will test negative for ketones and not match the ketone levels in your bloodstream as the body becomes more efficient at utilising ketones.

  Ketone breath meters and ketone blood meters can measure ketone levels and give you an accurate reading of ketone levels but are quite expensive compared to ketone test strips.

- You can re-enter ketosis using coconuts by having more coconut meat (doing coconut ketosis a second or third time) once you are already in ketosis.

I do not recommend using coconut oil on its own to re-enter ketosis as too much coconut oil has a laxative effect. Coconut meat, however, contains fibre that will keep your bowel movements steady and vitamins and minerals that help alkalise the body.

Each time you re-enter ketosis consecutively the effects of ketosis increase. I do not recommend entering ketosis more than three times in one session and make sure you keep an eye on your sodium and vitamin B12 levels. The body will lose sodium and vitamin B12 each time you enter ketosis.

Please do not try this if you are pregnant or while driving a vehicle due to the potential side effects of entering ketosis.

Coffee Ketosis

Please read all of the instructions before you begin.

What to do:

- Drink a double strength black coffee (or single strength if the coffee has double the caffeine content than standard coffee) and wait around 20 to 75 minutes to enter ketosis.

  Drink nothing but water (spring or distilled) during and after the process for at least 1 hour after you have entered ketosis.

Before you begin:

- Wait at least 30 to 60 minutes after a meal or drink (with the exception of water) before trying coffee ketosis as food in the colon can interfere with the process. Coffee ketosis works well first thing in the morning on an empty stomach.

You can do coffee ketosis right after a meal and enter ketosis 20 to 75 minutes later, but it does not always work after food and can be hit or miss. Waiting a while after a meal or drink will increase your chances of entering ketosis.

- You can mix other ingredients with the coffee such as milk and sugar as long as there is enough caffeine to trigger ketosis.

Adding half a teaspoon of cayenne and black pepper to a standard single strength coffee will get you into ketosis off half the recommended dose as cayenne pepper and black pepper increase the bioavailability, absorption and metabolism of caffeine found in coffee that triggers ketosis.

If you are not a fan of cayenne pepper, just use black pepper as it is the black pepper that allows you to have half the recommended dose to enter ketosis.

If you have never tried coffee ketosis before I do not recommend mixing the coffee with other ingredients initially, so you get an idea of what coffee ketosis is about.

- Do alone as the energy of others (including pets) can affect the process unless the others involved are not giving out negative energy or conditioning you and the process with their opinions or desires (subconscious or other-wise).

  If you live on a busy street, it may be a good idea to close the curtains or blinds to avoid others conditioning you. Emotions and thoughts are electrical in nature and have an effect on our neurochemistry. Avoid social media sites or contact with people via touch or technology and do not hold or wear any crystals/gems/metal jewellery or use a grounding mat or sheet as they can interfere with the process.

- If you have any medical conditions or are taking any medication, try coffee ketosis supervised initially to avoid any complications.

What to expect:

- Mental calm.
- No mental highs or lows.
- No blood sugar highs or lows.
- Improved eyesight.
- Increased mental concentration.

- Increased mental and physical energy.
- A balanced mind.
- Diminished appetite.
- An increase in breathing and a need for more air.
- No withdrawals or cravings for the things you were addicted to.

Typical symptoms of ketosis:
(include but not always).

- Cold shins and hands.
- Increased mental alertness.
- Increased concentration and focus.
- Tense shoulders.
- Feeling limber/supple joints.
- Increased strength in the legs and spinal column.
- Occasional mental calmness.
- Tears (for first timers only but not always).
- An increase in confidence.
- Feeling thirsty.
- Slight nausea.
- Bad breath (ketone breath).
- Tongue sticking to the roof of your mouth.
- Feeling angry/stressed/emotional (due to the release of toxins).
- Increased sense of smell.
- Horrible taste in your mouth from ketones.

- Runny nose (keto flu).

What to consider:

- If this is your first-time entering ketosis and you have lived a very toxic lifestyle, when you enter ketosis, you may cry as toxins are released into the bloodstream. Tears are one way the body releases toxins. This is fine and nothing to worry about as entering ketosis breaks down body fat where toxins are stored.

- Have plenty of sodium, around 4000 - 7000mg (about 2 - 3 teaspoons/15 - 18g of salt) the day before and/or on the day. Ketosis releases sodium from the kidneys as it lowers insulin levels in the body, the hormone that regulates blood sugar levels and appetite.

  If you eat a standard western diet sodium is not something to worry about, but if you eat a low sodium diet, a little extra sodium will help. The body's sodium requirements increase when you follow a ketogenic diet or enter ketosis regularly.

  Sometimes it is common to crave salty junk food after entering ketosis, but it is the sodium the body craves that is in the junk food and not the junk food per se. If you crave salty food after you have entered ketosis then you have not had enough sodium prior to entering ketosis. Eat something high in sodium to satisfy the cravings for salty food.

Good sources of sodium:

— Sea salt (2338mg per 6g).
— Himalayan salt (1080mg per 6g).
— Sea vegetables - Seaweed, Algae (Kombu highest @ 2727mg per 100g).
— Samphire (2500mg per 100g).
— Beet greens (226mg per 100g).
— Swiss chard (213mg per 100g).
— Celery (80mg per 100g).

• If you have anything that once caused an addiction after entering ketosis, it will restart the cycle of addiction again to the substance that you were addicted to by altering the chemistry of the brain and disrupting homeostasis. You will need to enter ketosis again to stop the cycle of addiction and reset the chemistry of the brain/gut flora.

We become addicted to things because those substances whether they are food or drugs alter our neurochemistry and as a result, our bodies crave such substances to readdress the chemical imbalance within and return to homeostasis. We can however, control our substance/food use while in ketosis for example if we had an addiction to alcohol/junk food where we binged to the point of excess (when out of ketosis), while in ketosis we can have one beer or packet of crisps and leave it at that, but if we get out of ketosis by going over the carbohydrate threshold (beer and crisps both being carbohydrates) it will start the binge cycle of addiction again and cravings will compel us to have more beer or crisps until we enter ketosis again to stop the cycle of addiction/cravings.

I have found that bingeing only happens again when we have not been abstinent for a long period of time as our brains and neural networks are still wired/programmed to binge. If we have been abstinent for years and are familiar with entering ketosis, the neural networks that supported our binge patterns of behaviour will no longer exist as our tolerance to substances is a direct result of how many neural networks we have built up over the years.

Ketosis allows us to have the substances we were once addicted to in a controlled manner if we remain in ketosis or re-enter ketosis. Ketosis gives us the freedom to choose when and what to consume in a way that suits us as ketosis gives us the freedom over food and substances when our nutritional needs are met. Some people only eat one meal a day (OMAD diet) as opposed to three main meals a day, and some people eat even less than that thanks to the power of ketosis (Inedia/Breatharians).

Once you have entered ketosis, you do not need to stay in ketosis for more than an hour for it to reset the chemistry of the brain/gut flora. After that it is up to you what to do. You can stay in ketosis if you like or get yourself out of ketosis by eating around 90 grams or more or carbohydrates in one sitting.

If you want to remain in ketosis keep your carbohydrate intake low (around 20 - 70g per day not including fibre). If you want to get in and out of ketosis throughout the day for whatever reason, the amount of carbohydrates you have throughout the day is irrelevant when you enter ketosis using coffee (unless you have an unusually high amount of carbohydrates throughout the day).

- Dose may vary depending on the quality and type of coffee used, whether or not you have the coffee cold, raw or in boiling water, your digestion, your body weight and what the coffee has been mixed with.

If coffee ketosis does not work the first-time experiment with a larger or smaller dose and/or add cayenne and black pepper the next time and see what works best for you, or alternatively use a different method to enter ketosis.

You may want to try coconut ketosis instead if you have an addiction to coffee/caffeine. If your addiction is to anything other than caffeine, coffee ketosis should work fine.

Additional information:

- For best results enter ketosis nutritionally and make sure you have eaten well the day before, and/or on the day to feel the full benefits of entering ketosis. Have plenty of citrus fruit as the citric acid in the fruit helps with the Krebs /Citric acid cycle and energy levels.

  Once ketosis sets in you should feel great and full of vigour. If you feel weak or low, it is because you have not addressed a nutritional deficiency that existed prior to entering ketosis. Ketosis will still work and reset the chemical set points of the body but should be followed up by meeting the body's nutritional needs i.e., a plant-based whole food alkaline diet.

- Raw (green) coffee beans are best, followed by boiled and then roasted but any coffee can be used depending on your preference. Unroasted green coffee cleanses the liver and colon due to its high vibrational energy and nutritional content. Raw coffee beans are minimally processed and contain live enzymes which ease the body's role of digesting and assimilating the nutrients found in coffee.

  I have not included the instructions for raw coffee as roasted coffee is convenient and easier to use and buy for most people than raw coffee.

- Coffee contains caffeine which is a drug. Too much caffeine has a laxative effect and can cause health problems. Coffee can be very acidic if used too often and can deplete the body of vitamins and minerals.

- Entering ketosis uses up reserves of sodium and vitamin B12 so be sure to have plenty if you enter ketosis on a regular basis. Be sure to have at least 4000 - 7000mg of sodium per day (about 2 - 3 teaspoons/15 - 18g of salt).

The Hydroxocobalamin or Methylcobalamin forms of vitamin B12 are the best bioavailable forms of B12 to use as they have the highest absorption rate. I recommend taking a high strength Methyl-cobalamin (vitamin B12) sublingual supplement of 1000mcg or more (daily) if you enter ketosis on a regular basis.

If you get pins and needles (a numbing of the fingers and toes) after entering ketosis it is a sign of vitamin B12 deficiency, so be sure to get your vitamin B12 levels checked at the doctors and supplement immediately.

Use a good quality sea salt or rock salt such as Himalayan salt or a natural unrefined sea salt (free from anti-caking agents). Table salt has been linked to health problems such as high blood pressure, kidney disease and an increased risk of heart attacks.

- Do not use tap water as tap water contains pollut-ants and contaminants that are harmful to our health. Tap water contains endocrine disruptors, hormones, plastics, pesticides, heavy metals, medications, nitrates and fertilisers.

The pollutants found in tap water have been found to cause neurological disorders and have been linked to hormonal disruptions, cancer and Alzheimer's disease. Use a good quality water such as spring or distilled water that does not contain the harmful impurities found in tap water.

- The best way to tell if you have entered ketosis is to see if your tongue is sticking to the roof of your mouth and you have an increased need for air. You may also notice an improvement in concentration, focus, eyesight and sense of smell.

  If you are unsure whether you have entered ketosis buy some ketone test strips and test your urine for ketones 2 - 6 hours after entering ketosis or first thing in the morning the following day.

  After following a ketogenic diet for a while and/or entering ketosis regularly, the ketone test strips will test negative for ketones and not match the ketone levels in your bloodstream as the body becomes more efficient at utilising ketones.

  Ketone breath meters and ketone blood meters can measure ketone levels and give you an accurate reading of ketone levels but are quite expensive compared to ketone test strips.

- You can re-enter ketosis using coffee by having more coffee (doing coffee ketosis a second or third time) once you are already in ketosis.

  Use a good quality coffee with a high caffeine content such as Arabica or Robusta or use a standard strength spiced coffee to re-enter ketosis as these types of coffee seem to get you into ketosis quicker than a standard coffee.

  Each time you re-enter ketosis consecutively the effects of ketosis increase. I do not recommend entering ketosis more than three times in one session and make sure you keep an eye on your sodium and vitamin B12 levels. The body will lose sodium and vitamin B12 each time you enter ketosis.

Please do not try this if you are pregnant or while driving a vehicle due to the potential side effects of entering ketosis.

Cacao Ketosis

Please read all of the instructions before you begin.

What to do:

- Take 84g of cacao in one go either in a smoothie or mousse or by eating it in bar or bean form and wait around 20 to 45 minutes to enter ketosis.

  Drink nothing but water (spring or distilled) during and after the process for at least 1 hour after you have entered ketosis.

Before you begin:

- Wait at least 30 to 60 minutes after a meal or drink (with the exception of water) before trying cacao ketosis as food in the colon can interfere with the process. Cacao ketosis works well first thing in the morning on an empty stomach.

- You can mix other ingredients with the cacao (to make chocolate bars, mousses, etc.) to make it taste better as long as there is at least 84g of cacao for it to work and no more than 60 - 80g of sugar in total but this may differ for each of us.

  Store-bought dark chocolate with a high cacao content works that contains other ingredients such as unrefined sugar and flavourings.

  Adding half a teaspoon of cayenne and black pepper to the cacao will get you into ketosis off half the recommended dose (42g) as cayenne and black pepper increase the bioavailability, absorption and metabolism of caffeine found in cacao that triggers ketosis.

  If you are not a fan of cayenne pepper, just use black pepper as it is the black pepper that allows you to have half the recommended dose to enter ketosis and be sure to reduce the sugar content respectively if spices are used in the recipe to 30 - 40g of sugar in total including the sugars naturally found in food.

  Make sure you use a good quality cacao product as the quality of the cacao is very important as some cacao powders give you really bad stomach-ache and make you feel unwell.

If you have never tried cacao ketosis before I do not recommend mixing the cacao with other ingredients initially so you get an idea of what cacao ketosis is about.

- Do alone as the energy of others (including pets) can affect the process unless the others involved are not giving out negative energy or conditioning you and the process with their opinions or desires (subconscious or otherwise).

  If you live on a busy street, it may be a good idea to close the curtains or blinds to avoid others conditioning you. Emotions and thoughts are electrical in nature and have an effect on our neurochemistry. Avoid social media sites or contact with people via touch or technology and do not hold or wear any crystals/gems/metal jewellery or use a grounding mat or sheet as they can interfere with the process.

- If you have any medical conditions or are taking any medication, try cacao ketosis supervised initially to avoid any complications.

What to expect:

- Mental calm.
- No mental highs or lows.
- No blood sugar highs or lows.
- Improved eyesight.
- Increased mental concentration.
- Increased mental and physical energy.
- A balanced mind.
- Diminished appetite.
- An increase in breathing and a need for more air.
- No withdrawals or cravings for the things you were addicted to.

Typical symptoms of ketosis:
(include but not always).

- Cold shins and hands.
- Increased mental alertness.
- Increased concentration and focus.
- Tense shoulders.
- Feeling limber/supple joints.
- Increased strength in the legs and spinal column.
- Occasional mental calmness.
- Tears (for first timers only but not always).
- An increase in confidence.
- Feeling thirsty.

- Slight nausea.
- Bad breath (ketone breath).
- Tongue sticking to the roof of your mouth.
- Feeling angry/stressed/emotional (due to the release of toxins).
- Increased sense of smell.
- Horrible taste in your mouth from ketones.
- Stomach-ache (cacao draws toxins from your stomach/intestines).
- Runny nose (keto flu).

What to consider:

- If this is your first-time entering ketosis and you have lived a very toxic lifestyle, when you enter ketosis, you may cry as toxins are released into the bloodstream. Tears are one way the body releases toxins. This is fine and nothing to worry about as entering ketosis breaks down body fat where toxins are stored.

- Have plenty of sodium, around 4000 - 7000mg (about 2 - 3 teaspoons/15 - 18g of salt) the day before and/or on the day. Ketosis releases sodium from the kidneys as it lowers insulin levels in the body, the hormone that regulates blood sugar levels and appetite.

If you eat a standard western diet sodium is not something to worry about, but if you eat a low sodium diet, a little extra sodium will help. The body's sodium requirements increase when you follow a ketogenic diet or enter ketosis regularly.

Sometimes it is common to crave salty junk food after entering ketosis, but it is the sodium the body craves that is in the junk food and not the junk food per se. If you crave salty food after you have entered ketosis then you have not had enough sodium prior to entering ketosis. Eat something high in sodium to satisfy the cravings for salty food.

Good sources of sodium:

— Sea salt (2338mg per 6g).
— Himalayan salt (1080mg per 6g).
— Sea vegetables - Seaweed, Algae (Kombu highest @ 2727mg per 100g).
— Samphire (2500mg per 100g).
— Beet greens (226mg per 100g).
— Swiss chard (213mg per 100g).
— Celery (80mg per 100g).

• If you have anything that once caused an addiction after entering ketosis, it will restart the cycle of addiction again to the substance that you were addicted to by altering the chemistry of the brain and disrupting homeostasis. You will need to enter ketosis again to stop the cycle of addiction and reset the chemistry of the brain/gut flora.

We become addicted to things because those substances whether they are food or drugs alter our neurochemistry and as a result, our bodies crave such substances to readdress the chemical imbalance within and return to homeostasis. We can however, control our substance/food use while in ketosis for example if we had an addiction to alcohol/junk food where we binged to the point of excess (when out of ketosis), while in ketosis we can have one beer or packet of crisps and leave it at that, but if we get out of ketosis by going over the carbohydrate threshold (beer and crisps both being carbohydrates) it will start the binge cycle of addiction again and cravings will compel us to have more beer or crisps until we enter ketosis again to stop the cycle of addiction/cravings.

I have found that bingeing only happens again when we have not been abstinent for a long period of time as our brains and neural networks are still wired/programmed to binge. If we have been abstinent for years and are familiar with entering ketosis, the neural networks that supported our binge patterns of behaviour will no longer exist as our tolerance to substances is a direct result of how many neural networks we have built up over the years.

Ketosis allows us to have the substances we were once addicted to in a controlled manner if we remain in ketosis or re-enter ketosis. Ketosis gives us the freedom to choose when and what to consume in a way that suits us as ketosis gives us the freedom over food and substances when our nutritional needs are met. Some people only eat one meal a day (OMAD diet) as opposed to three main meals a day, and some people eat even less than that thanks to the power of ketosis (Inedia/ Breatharians).

Once you have entered ketosis, you do not need to stay in ketosis for more than an hour for it to reset the chemistry of the brain/gut flora. After that it is up to you what to do. You can stay in ketosis if you like or get yourself out of ketosis by eating around 90 grams or more of carbohydrates in one sitting.

If you want to remain in ketosis keep your carbohydrate intake low (around 20 - 70g per day not including fibre). If you want to get in and out of ketosis throughout the day for whatever reason, the amount of carbohydrates you have throughout the day is irrelevant when you enter ketosis using cacao (unless you have an unusually high amount of carbohydrates throughout the day).

- Dose may vary depending on the quality and type of cacao used, whether the cacao has been cooked or not, your body weight, your digestion and what the cacao has been mixed with.

If cacao ketosis does not work the first-time experiment with a larger or smaller dose and/or add cayenne and black pepper the next time and see what works best for you, or alternatively use a different method to enter ketosis.

You may want to try coconut ketosis instead if you have an addiction to cacao/caffeine. If your addiction is to anything other than cacao/caffeine, cacao ketosis should work fine.

Additional information:

- For best results enter ketosis nutritionally and make sure you have eaten well the day before, and/or on the day to feel the full benefits of entering ketosis. Have plenty of citrus fruit as the citric acid in the fruit helps with the Krebs /Citric acid cycle and energy levels.

Once ketosis sets in you should feel great and full of vigour. If you feel weak or low, it is because you have not addressed a nutritional deficiency that existed prior to entering ketosis. Ketosis will still work and reset the chemical set points of the body but should be followed up by meeting the body's nutritional needs i.e., a plant-based whole food alkaline diet.

- Raw cacao is best, followed by cooked cacao but any cacao can be used depending on your preference. Drinking chocolate (cocoa) can be used too but drinking chocolate is usually heavily processed and devoid of nutrients. If you prefer to have a hot or cold chocolate drink, make it from raw or cooked cacao powder.

  Raw cacao cleanses the liver and colon due to its high vibrational energy and nutritional content. Raw cacao is minimally processed and contains live enzymes which ease the body's role of digesting and assimilating the nutrients we get from cacao.

- Cacao contains caffeine and theobromine which are drugs. Too much caffeine and theobromine have a laxative effect and can cause health problems. Cacao can be very acidic if used too often and can deplete the body of vitamins and minerals.

- Entering ketosis uses up reserves of sodium and vitamin B12 so be sure to have plenty if you enter ketosis on a regular basis. Be sure to have at least 4000 - 7000mg of sodium per day (about 2 - 3 teaspoons/15 - 18g of salt).

The Hydroxocobalamin or Methylcobalamin forms of vitamin B12 are the best bioavailable forms of B12 to use as they have the highest absorption rate. I recommend taking a high strength Methylcobalamin (vitamin B12) sublingual supplement of 1000mcg or more (daily) if you enter ketosis on a regular basis.

If you get pins and needles (a numbing of the fingers and toes) after entering ketosis it is a sign of vitamin B12 deficiency, so be sure to get your vitamin B12 levels checked at the doctors and supplement immediately.

Use a good quality sea salt or rock salt such as Himalayan salt or a natural unrefined sea salt (free from anti-caking agents). Table salt has been linked to health problems such as high blood pressure, kidney disease and an increased risk of heart attacks.

- Do not use tap water as tap water contains pollutants and contaminants that are harmful to our health. Tap water contains endocrine disruptors, hormones, plastics, pesticides, heavy metals, medications, nitrates and fertilisers.

  The pollutants found in tap water have been found to cause neurological disorders and have been linked to hormonal disruptions, cancer and Alzheimer's disease. Use a good quality water such as spring or distilled water that does not contain the harmful impurities found in tap water.

- The best way to tell if you have entered ketosis is to see if your tongue is sticking to the roof of your mouth and you have an increased need for air. You may also notice an improvement in concentration, focus, eyesight and sense of smell.

  If you are unsure whether you have entered ketosis buy some ketone test strips and test your urine for ketones 2 - 6 hours after entering ketosis or first thing in the morning the following day.

  After following a ketogenic diet for a while and/or entering ketosis regularly, the ketone test strips will test negative for ketones and not match the ketone levels in your bloodstream as the body becomes more efficient at utilising ketones.

Ketone breath meters and ketone blood meters can measure ketone levels and give you an accurate reading of ketone levels but are quite expensive compared to ketone test strips.

- You can re-enter ketosis using cacao by having more cacao (doing cacao ketosis a second or third time) once you are already in ketosis. Use black pepper with the cacao so you do not need to use as much cacao to re-enter ketosis.

Each time you re-enter ketosis consecutively the effects of ketosis increase. I do not recommend entering ketosis more than three times in one session and make sure you keep an eye on your sodium and vitamin B12 levels. The body will lose sodium and vitamin B12 each time you enter ketosis.

Please do not try this if you are pregnant or while driving a vehicle due to the potential side effects of entering ketosis.

Tea Ketosis

Please read all of the instructions before you begin.

What to do:

- Drink a double strength black tea (2 standard tea bags brewed for about 5 minutes) and wait around 20 to 75 minutes to enter ketosis.

  Drink nothing but water (spring or distilled) during and after the process for at least 1 hour after you have entered ketosis.

Before you begin:

- Wait at least 30 to 60 minutes after a meal or drink (with the exception of water) before trying tea ketosis as food in the colon can interfere with the process. Tea ketosis works well first thing in the morning on an empty stomach.

  You can do tea ketosis right after a meal and enter ketosis 20 to 45 minutes later, but it does not always work after food and can be

57

hit or miss. Waiting a while after a meal or drink will increase your chances of entering ketosis.

- You can mix other ingredients with the tea such as milk and sugar as long as there is enough caffeine to trigger ketosis.

  Adding half a teaspoon of cayenne and black pepper to a standard single strength black tea will get you into ketosis off half the recommended dose as cayenne and black pepper increase the bioavailability, absorption and metabolism of caffeine found in tea that triggers ketosis.

  If you are not a fan of cayenne pepper, just use black pepper as it is the black pepper that allows you to have half the recommended dose to enter ketosis.

  If you have never tried tea ketosis before I do not recommend mixing the tea with other ingredients initially so you get an idea of what tea ketosis is about.

- Do alone as the energy of others (including pets) can affect the process unless the others involved are not giving out negative energy or conditioning you and the process with their opinions or desires (subconscious or otherwise).

If you live on a busy street, it may be a good idea to close the curtains or blinds to avoid others conditioning you. Emotions and thoughts are electrical in nature and have an effect on our neurochemistry. Avoid social media sites or contact with people via touch or technology, and do not hold or wear any crystals/gems/metal jewellery or use a grounding mat or sheet, as they can interfere with the process.

- If you have any medical conditions or are taking any medication, try tea ketosis super-vised initially to avoid any complications.

What to expect:

- Mental calm.
- No mental highs or lows.
- No blood sugar highs or lows.
- Improved eyesight.
- Increased mental concentration.
- Increased mental and physical energy.
- A balanced mind.
- Diminished appetite.
- An increase in breathing and a need for more air.
- No withdrawals or cravings for the things you were addicted to.

Typical symptoms of ketosis:
(include but not always).

- Cold shins and hands.
- Increased mental alertness.
- Increased concentration and focus.
- Tense shoulders.
- Feeling limber/supple joints.
- Increased strength in the legs and spinal column.
- Occasional mental calmness.
- Tears (for first timers only but not always).
- An increase in confidence.
- Feeling thirsty.
- Slight nausea.
- Bad breath (ketone breath).
- Tongue sticking to the roof of your mouth.
- Feeling angry/stressed/emotional (due to the release of toxins).
- Increased sense of smell.
- Horrible taste in your mouth from ketones.
- Runny nose (keto flu).

What to consider:

- If this is your first-time entering ketosis and you have lived a very toxic lifestyle, when you enter ketosis, you may cry as toxins are released into the bloodstream. Tears are one way the body releases toxins. This is fine and nothing to worry about as entering ketosis breaks down body fat where toxins are stored.

- Have plenty of sodium, around 4000 - 7000mg (about 2 - 3 teaspoons/15 - 18g of salt) the day before and/or on the day. Ketosis releases sodium from the kidneys as it lowers insulin levels in the body, the hormone that regulates blood sugar levels and appetite.

If you eat a standard western diet sodium is not something to worry about, but if you eat a low sodium diet, a little extra sodium will help. The body's sodium requirements increase when you follow a ketogenic diet or enter ketosis regularly.

Sometimes it is common to crave salty junk food after entering ketosis, but it is the sodium the body craves that is in the junk food and not the junk food per se. If you crave salty food after you have entered ketosis then you have not had enough sodium prior to entering ketosis. Eat something high in sodium to satisfy the cravings for salty food.

Good sources of sodium:

— Sea salt (2338mg per 6g).
— Himalayan Salt (1080mg per 6g).
— Sea vegetables - Seaweed, Algae (Kombu highest @ 2727mg per 100g).
— Samphire (2500mg per 100g).
— Beet greens (226mg per 100g).
— Swiss chard (213mg per 100g).
— Celery (80mg per 100g).

• If you have anything that once caused an addiction after entering ketosis, it will restart the cycle of addiction again to the substance that you were addicted to by altering the chemistry of the brain and disrupting homeostasis. You will need to enter ketosis again to stop the cycle of addiction and reset the chemistry of the brain/gut flora.

We become addicted to things because those substances whether they are food or drugs alter our neurochemistry and as a result, our bodies crave such substances to readdress the chemical imbalance within and return to homeostasis. We can however, control our substance/food use while in ketosis for example if we had an addiction to alcohol/junk food where we binged to the point of excess (when out of ketosis), while in ketosis we can have one beer or packet of crisps and leave it at that, but if we get out of ketosis by going over the carbohydrate threshold (beer and crisps both being carbohydrates) it will start the binge cycle of addiction again and cravings will compel us to have more beer or crisps until we enter ketosis again to stop the cycle of addiction/cravings.

I have found that bingeing only happens again when we have not been abstinent for a long period of time as our brains and neural networks are still wired/programmed to binge. If we have been abstinent for years and are familiar with entering ketosis, the neural networks that supported our binge patterns of behaviour will no longer exist as our tolerance to substances is a direct result of how many neural networks we have built up over the years.

Ketosis allows us to have the substances we were once addicted to in a controlled manner if we remain in ketosis or re-enter ketosis. Ketosis gives us the freedom to choose when and what to consume in a way that suits us as ketosis gives us the freedom over food and substances when our nutritional needs are met. Some people only eat one meal a day (OMAD diet) as opposed to three main meals a day, and some people eat even less than that thanks to the power of ketosis (Inedia/ Breatharians).

Once you have entered ketosis, you do not need to stay in ketosis for more than an hour for it to reset the chemistry of the brain/gut flora. After that it is up to you what to do. You can stay in ketosis if you like or get yourself out of ketosis by eating around 90 grams or more of carbohydrates in one sitting.

If you want to remain in ketosis keep your carbohydrate intake low (around 20 - 70g per day not including fibre). If you want to get in and out of ketosis throughout the day for whatever reason the amount of carbohydrates you have throughout the day is irrelevant when you enter ketosis using tea (unless you have an unusually high amount of carbohydrates throughout the day).

- Dose may vary depending on the quality and type of tea used, whether you have the tea cold, raw or in boiling water, your digestion, your body weight and what the tea has been mixed with.

If tea ketosis does not work the first-time experiment with a larger or smaller dose and/or add cayenne and black pepper the next time and see what works best for you, or alternatively use a different method to enter ketosis.

You may want to try coconut ketosis instead if you have an addiction to tea/caffeine. If your addiction is to anything other than caffeine, tea ketosis should work fine.

Additional information:

- For best results enter ketosis nutritionally and make sure you have eaten well the day before, and/or on the day to feel the full benefits of entering ketosis. Have plenty of citrus fruit as the citric acid in the fruit helps with the Krebs/ Citric acid cycle and energy levels.

  Once ketosis sets in you should feel great and full of vigour. If you feel weak or low, it is because you have not addressed a nutritional deficiency that existed prior to entering ketosis. Ketosis will still work and reset the chemical set points of the body but should be followed up by meeting the body's nutritional needs i.e., a plant-based whole food alkaline diet.

- Raw tea is best, but cooked or brewed tea can be used depending on your preference. Raw tea cleanses the liver and colon due to its high vibrational energy and nutritional content. Raw tea is minimally processed and contains live enzymes which ease the body's role of digesting and assimilating the nutrients we get from tea.

- Tea contains caffeine which is a drug. Too much caffeine has a laxative effect and can cause health problems. Tea can be acidic if used too often and can deplete the body of vitamins and minerals.

- Entering ketosis uses up reserves of sodium and vitamin B12 so be sure to have plenty if you enter ketosis on a regular basis. Be sure to have at least 4000 - 7000mg of sodium per day (about 2 - 3 teaspoons/15 - 18g of salt).

The Hydroxocobalamin or Methylcobalamin forms of vitamin B12 are the best bioavailable forms of B12 to use as they have the highest absorption rate. I recommend taking a high strength Methylcobalamin (vitamin B12) sublingual supplement of 1000mcg or more (daily) if you enter ketosis on a regular basis.

If you get pins and needles (a numbing of the fingers and toes) after entering ketosis it is a sign of vitamin B12 deficiency, so be sure to get your vitamin B12 levels checked at the doctors and supplement immediately.

Use a good quality sea salt or rock salt such as Himalayan salt or a natural unrefined sea salt (free from anti-caking agents). Table salt has been linked to health problems such as high blood pressure, kidney disease and an increased risk of heart attacks.

- Do not use tap water as tap water contains pollutants and contaminants that are harmful to our health. Tap water contains endocrine disruptors, hormones, plastics, pesticides, heavy metals, medications, nitrates and fertilisers.

  The pollutants found in tap water have been found to cause neurological disorders and have been linked to hormonal disruptions, cancer and Alzheimer's disease. Use a good quality water such as spring or distilled water that does not contain the harmful impurities found in tap water.

- The best way to tell if you have entered ketosis is to see if your tongue is sticking to the roof of your mouth and you have an increased need for air. You may also notice an improvement in concentration, focus, eyesight and sense of smell.

If you are unsure whether you have entered ketosis buy some ketone test strips and test your urine for ketones 2 - 6 hours after entering ketosis or first thing in the morning the following day.

After following a ketogenic diet for a while and/or entering ketosis regularly, the ketone test strips will test negative for ketones and not match the ketone levels in your blood-stream as the body becomes more efficient at utilising ketones.

Ketone breath meters and ketone blood meters can measure ketone levels and give you an accurate reading of ketone levels but are quite expensive compared to ketone test strips.

- You can re-enter ketosis using tea by having more tea (doing tea ketosis a second or third time) once you are already in ketosis.

Each time you re-enter ketosis consecutively the effects of ketosis increase. I do not recommend entering ketosis more than three times in one session and make sure you keep an eye on your sodium and vitamin B12 levels. The body will lose sodium and vitamin B12 each time you enter ketosis.

Please do not try this if you are pregnant or while driving a vehicle due to the potential side effects of entering ketosis.

Matcha Ketosis

Please read all of the instructions before you begin.

What to do:

- Take 0.3g of matcha powder (about 1/8th of a teaspoon) with a cup of water and wait around 20 to 45 minutes to enter ketosis.

  Drink nothing but water (spring or distilled) during and after the process for at least 1 hour after you have entered ketosis.

Before you begin:

- Wait at least 30 to 60 minutes after a meal or drink (with the exception of water) before trying matcha ketosis as food in the colon can interfere with the process. Matcha ketosis works well first thing in the morning on an empty stomach.

You can do matcha ketosis right after a meal and enter ketosis 20 to 45 minutes later, but it does not always work after food and can be hit or miss. Waiting a while after a meal or drink will increase your chances of entering ketosis.

- You can mix other ingredients with the matcha such as milk and sugar as long as there is enough caffeine to trigger ketosis.

  Adding half a teaspoon of cayenne and black pepper to matcha will get you into ketosis off half the recommended dose (0.15 grams) as cayenne and black pepper increase the bioavailability, absorption and metabolism of caffeine found in matcha that triggers ketosis.

  If you are not a fan of cayenne pepper, just use black pepper as it is the black pepper that allows you to have half the recommended dose to enter ketosis.

  If you have never tried matcha ketosis before I do not recommend mixing the matcha with other ingredients initially, so you get an idea of what matcha ketosis is about.

- Do alone as the energy of others (including pets) can affect the process unless the others involved are not giving out negative energy or conditioning you and the process with their opinions or desires (subconscious or other-wise).

  If you live on a busy street, it may be a good idea to close the curtains or blinds to avoid others conditioning you. Emotions and thoughts are electrical in nature and have an effect on our neurochemistry. Avoid social media sites or contact with people via touch or technology, and do not hold or wear any crystals/gems/metal jewellery or use a grounding mat or sheet, as they can interfere with the process.

- If you have any medical conditions or are taking any medication, try matcha ketosis supervised initially to avoid any complications.

What to expect:

- Mental calm.
- No mental highs or lows.
- No blood sugar highs or lows.
- Improved eyesight.
- Increased mental concentration.

- Increased mental and physical energy.
- A balanced mind.
- Diminished appetite.
- An increase in breathing and a need for more air.
- No withdrawals or cravings for the things you were addicted to.

Typical symptoms of ketosis:
(include but not always).

- Cold shins and hands.
- Increased mental alertness.
- Increased concentration and focus.
- Tense shoulders.
- Feeling limber/supple joints.
- Increased strength in the legs and spinal column.
- Occasional mental calmness.
- Tears (for first timers only but not always).
- An increase in confidence.
- Feeling thirsty.
- Slight nausea.
- Bad breath (ketone breath).
- Tongue sticking to the roof of your mouth.
- Feeling angry/stressed/emotional (due to the release of toxins).
- Increased sense of smell.
- Horrible taste in your mouth from ketones.

- Runny nose (keto flu).

What to consider:

- If this is your first-time entering ketosis and you have lived a very toxic lifestyle, when you enter ketosis, you may cry as toxins are released into the bloodstream. Tears are one way the body releases toxins. This is fine and nothing to worry about as entering ketosis breaks down body fat where toxins are stored.

- Have plenty of sodium, around 4000 - 7000mg (about 2 - 3 teaspoons/15 - 18g of salt) the day before and/or on the day. Ketosis releases sodium from the kidneys as it lowers insulin levels in the body, the hormone that regulates blood sugar levels and appetite.

  If you eat a standard western diet sodium is not something to worry about, but if you eat a low sodium diet, a little extra sodium will help. The body's sodium requirements increase when you follow a ketogenic diet or enter ketosis regularly.

  Sometimes it is common to crave salty junk food after entering ketosis, but it is the sodium the body craves that is in the junk food and not the junk food per se. If you crave salty food after you have entered ketosis then you have not had enough sodium prior to entering ketosis. Eat something high in sodium to satisfy the cravings for salty food.

Good sources of sodium:

- Sea salt (2338mg per 6g).
- Himalayan Salt (1080mg per 6g).
- Sea vegetables - Seaweed, Algae (Kombu highest @ 2727mg per 100g).
- Samphire (2500mg per 100g).
- Beet greens (226mg per 100g).
- Swiss chard (213mg per 100g).
- Celery (80mg per 100g).

• If you have anything that once caused an addiction after entering ketosis, it will restart the cycle of addiction again to the substance that you were addicted to by altering the chemistry of the brain and disrupting homeostasis. You will need to enter ketosis again to stop the cycle of addiction and reset the chemistry of the brain/gut flora.

We become addicted to things because those substances whether they are food or drugs alter our neurochemistry and as a result, our bodies crave such substances to readdress the chemical imbalance within and return to homeostasis. We can however, control our substance/food use while in ketosis for example if we had an addiction to alcohol/junk food where we binged to the point of excess (when out of ketosis), while in ketosis we can have one beer or packet of crisps and leave it at that, but if we get out of ketosis by going over the carbohydrate threshold (beer and crisps both being carbohydrates) it will start the binge cycle of addiction again and cravings will compel us to have more beer or crisps until we enter ketosis again to stop the cycle of addiction/cravings.

I have found that bingeing only happens again when we haven't been abstinent for a long period of time as our brains and neural networks are still wired/programmed to binge. If we have been abstinent for years and are familiar with entering ketosis, the neural networks that supported our binge patterns of behaviour will no longer exist as our tolerance to substances is a direct result of how many neural networks we have built up over the years.

Ketosis allows us to have the substances we were once addicted to in a controlled manner if we remain in ketosis or re-enter ketosis. Ketosis gives us the freedom to choose when and what to consume in a way that suits us as ketosis gives us the freedom over food and substances when our nutritional needs are met. Some people only eat one meal a day (OMAD diet) as opposed to three main meals a day, and some people eat even less than that thanks to the power of ketosis (Inedia/ Breatharians).

Once you have entered ketosis, you do not need to stay in ketosis for more than an hour for it to reset the chemistry of the brain/gut flora. After that it is up to you what to do. You can stay in ketosis if you like or get yourself out of ketosis by eating around 90 grams or more of carbohydrates in one sitting.

If you want to remain in ketosis keep your carbohydrate intake low (around 20 - 70g per day not including fibre). If you want to get in and out of ketosis throughout the day for whatever reason the amount of carbohydrates you have throughout the day is irrelevant when you enter ketosis using matcha (unless you have an unusually high amount of carbohydrates throughout the day).

- Dose may vary depending on the quality and type of matcha used, whether you have the matcha cold, raw or in boiling water, your digestion, your body weight and what the matcha has been mixed with.

  If matcha ketosis does not work the first-time experiment with a larger or smaller dose and/or add cayenne and black pepper the next time and see what works best for you, or alternatively use a different method to enter ketosis.

  You may want to try coconut ketosis instead if you have an addiction to matcha/caffeine. If your addiction is to anything other than caffeine, matcha ketosis should work fine.

Additional information:

- For best results enter ketosis nutritionally and make sure you have eaten well the day before, and/or on the day to feel the full benefits of entering ketosis. Have plenty of citrus fruit as the citric acid in the fruit helps with the Krebs/Citric acid cycle and energy levels.

Once ketosis sets in you should feel great and full of vigour. If you feel weak or low, it is because you have not addressed a nutritional deficiency that existed prior to entering ketosis. Ketosis will still work and reset the chemical set points of the body but should be followed up by meeting the body's nutritional needs i.e., a plant-based whole food alkaline diet.

- Raw matcha is best, but cooked or brewed matcha can be used too depending on your preference. Raw matcha cleanses the liver and colon due to its high vibrational energy and nutritional content. Raw matcha is minimally processed and contains live enzymes which ease the body's role of digesting and assimilating the nutrients we get from matcha.

- Matcha contains caffeine which is a drug and too much can cause health problems. Too much matcha has a laxative effect and can deplete the body of vitamins and minerals.

- Entering ketosis uses up reserves of sodium and vitamin B12 so be sure to have plenty if you enter ketosis on a regular basis. Be sure to have at least 4000 - 7000mg of sodium per day (about 2 - 3 teaspoons/15 - 18g of salt).

The Hydroxocobalamin or Methylcobalamin forms of vitamin B12 are the best bioavailable forms of B12 to use as they have the highest absorption rate. I recommend taking a high strength Methylcobalamin (vitamin B12) sublingual supplement of 1000mcg or more (daily) if you enter ketosis on a regular basis.

If you get pins and needles (a numbing of the fingers and toes) after entering ketosis it is a sign of vitamin B12 deficiency, so be sure to get your vitamin B12 levels checked at the doctors and supplement immediately.

Use a good quality sea salt or rock salt such as Himalayan salt or a natural unrefined sea salt (free from anti-caking agents). Table salt has been linked to health problems such as high blood pressure, kidney disease and an increased risk of heart attacks.

- Do not use tap water as tap water contains pollutants and contaminants that are harmful to our health. Tap water contains endocrine disruptors, hormones, plastics, pesticides, heavy metals, medications, nitrates and fertilisers.

The pollutants found in tap water have been found to cause neurological disorders and have been linked to hormonal disruptions, cancer and Alzheimer's disease. Use a good quality water such as spring or distilled water that does not contain the harmful impurities found in tap water.

- The best way to tell if you have entered ketosis is to see if your tongue is sticking to the roof of your mouth and you have an increased need for air. You may also notice an improvement in concentration, focus, eyesight and sense of smell.

  If you are unsure whether you have entered ketosis buy some ketone test strips and test your urine for ketones 2 - 6 hours after entering ketosis or first thing in the morning the following day.

  After following a ketogenic diet for a while and/or entering ketosis regularly, the ketone test strips will test negative for ketones and not match the ketone levels in your bloodstream as the body becomes more efficient at utilising ketones.

  Ketone breath meters and ketone blood meters can measure ketone levels and give you an accurate reading of ketone levels but are quite expensive compared to ketone test strips.

- You can re-enter ketosis using matcha by having more matcha (doing matcha ketosis a second or third time) once you are already in ketosis.

  Matcha is a great way to re-enter ketosis as matcha is alkalising, packed with nutrients and has over 100 times the amount of antioxidants as green tea.

  Each time you re-enter ketosis consecutively the effects of ketosis increase. I do not recommend entering ketosis more than three times in one session and make sure you keep an eye on your sodium and vitamin B12 levels. The body will lose vitamin B12 and sodium each time you enter ketosis.

Please do not try this if you are pregnant or while driving a vehicle due to the potential side effects of entering ketosis.

Testimonials

Nicotine Addiction - Gaby, 25, Macclesfield.

I quit smoking by trying coconut ketosis after 6 years of being a smoker. My grandma had suffered from lung cancer through smoking and being a singer myself I knew how detrimental it was for my health and my career.

I tried so many different methods to quit from vaping, chewing gum, downloading apps and going cold turkey, but the intense withdrawals and anger that came with cutting out the nicotine made me hate myself and my behaviour, and I would smoke again just to feel normal.

When I tried coconut ketosis, I could not believe that something so simple had been the answer the whole time, and why no one was talking about it! My withdrawals, cravings and anger were gone, it was like the biggest weight had been lifted off me and for once I could finally move forward and ditch the smoking for good - with nothing holding me back!

Sugar Addiction - Mandy, 57, California.

I have always had a severe addiction to sugar. Being Type 1 diabetic (adult-onset at age 31), I would try to force myself to not have sugar but would ALWAYS sneak something in and have to shoot up extra insulin for it.

I have been doing Vegan Keto diet for 3 months now and have been in ketosis the whole time. I've lost 14 lbs, but the HUGE thing is that I have not eaten 1 sweet thing in 3 months and have no craving for it. I instinctively reach for cookies etc, out of habit, but then realize I don't actually crave it. I am also taking ⅓ the insulin I used to have on carb meals (excluding the extra I took for sugar cheats). Ketosis has also made me less hungry, so my meal sizes have shrunk drastically. Best thing that has ever happened to me!

Nicotine Addiction - Alexandra, 26, Manchester.

When I found out about coconut ketosis, I had a couple of doubts, kind of thought it was too good to be true to be honest because prior to trying it, I'd tried everything to quit and I just couldn't do it.

After 4 years of going back and forth trying to quit, coconut ketosis was my saviour. It worked!! It really works. I genuinely could not believe it. Especially because I never felt any withdrawals. It made me feel more in control and better within myself. I also do regular three-day water fasts and found it to be the perfect assistant alongside the coconut ketosis. It's truly amazing that there is no limit to how many times you can do coconut ketosis too!! Literally life-changing!! For that, I literally am beyond grateful.

Final Word

Now that we understand addiction from a neuro-chemical point of view, we have the means to stop the cycle of addiction in its tracks and live a life free from addiction.

We can now have the things that we were once addicted to in moderation in a controlled manner without bingeing to the point of excess through the power of ketosis and its ability to alter our neuro-chemistry in a beneficial way.

Addictions are not a sign of weakness but a sign that we have conditioned our bodies to want and depend on the things that mimic our internal chemistry.

I have found that ketosis can pick us up when we are feeling low and bring us down when we are too high as entering into ketosis cancels the effects that drink or drugs have on us.

Ketosis is our inner healer that can treat a number of mental and physical conditions and further research is needed on what other illnesses ketosis can alleviate as a lot of the scientific studies done have been carried out on animals and/or based on a ketogenic diet that includes animal products.

I urge you to be your own scientist and to test ketosis out for yourself as ketosis may heal or improve other conditions or illnesses that I have not had, mentioned or come across yet.

Ketosis is a great tool for any doctor, shaman, alchemist or health and fitness practitioner as the benefits of entering ketosis are vast. Ketosis can also be used to improve athletic performance and enhance spiritual practices such as prayer, reiki and meditation.

Ketosis is truly a gift from God that gives us the ability to control our cravings and is one of the many medicinal tools that we have at our disposal to help prevent and treat illnesses along with juicing, fasting, plant-based medicines, plant-based diets, pharmaceuticals and nutritional supplements.

The possibilities are endless when we combine a plant-based diet with the power of ketosis!

References

What is Addiction?

Addiction. (n.d.). In *Merriam-Webster.* Retrieved from
https://www.merriam-webster.com/dictionary/addiction?

American Psychiatric Association. (2017, January). *What Is
Addiction?* Retrieved from https://www.psychiatry.org
/patients-families/addiction/what-is-addiction

Koob, G. F., Arends, M. A., & Le, M. M. (2014). *Drugs,
Addiction, and the Brain*. Oxford: Academic Press -Elsevier.

Hesse M. (2006). What does addiction mean to me. *Mens
sana monographs, 4 (1),* 104–126.

Rinn, W., Desai, N., Rosenblatt, H., & Gastfriend, D. R. (2002).
Addiction denial and cognitive dysfunction: a preliminary
investigation. *The Journal of neuropsychiatry and clinical
neurosciences*, 14 (1), 52-57.

Moss, M. (2014). *Salt, Sugar, Fat: How the food giants hooked
us*. Random House UK.

Kennett, J. M., Matthews, S., & Snoek, A. (2013). Pleasure and
addiction. *Frontiers in psychiatry, 4,* 117.

Littleton J. (1998). Neurochemical mechanisms underlying
alcohol withdrawal. *Alcohol health and research world*,
22 (1), 13–24.

Extein, I. L., & Gold, M. S. (1993). Hypothesized neurochemical models for psychiatric syndromes in alcohol and drug dependence. *Journal of Addictive Diseases*, *12* (3), 29-43.

American Addiction Centre. (2019, June 17.) *Drug Abuse and Chemical Imbalance in the Brain: Dopamine, Serotonin & More*. Retrieved from https://americanaddictioncenters. org/health-complications-addiction/chemical-imbalance.

Aubele, T., Wenck, S., & Reynolds, S. (2011). *Train your brain to get happy: The simple program that primes your gray cells for joy, optimism, and serenity*. Avon, Mass: Adams Media.

Breuning, L. G. (2016). *Habits of a happy brain: Retrain your brain to boost your serotonin, dopamine, oxytocin, & endorphin levels*. Avon, Massachusetts: Adams Media.

Dfarhud, Dariush et al. "Happiness & Health: The Biological Factors- Systematic Review Article." *Iranian journal of public health* vol. 43,11 (2014): 1468-77.

Uvnas-Moberg, K., & Petersson, M. (2005). Oxytocin, a mediator of anti-stress, well-being, social interaction, growth and healing. *Z Psychosom Med Psychother,* 51 (1), 57-80.

Koob G. F. (2008). Hedonic Homeostatic Dysregulation as a Driver of Drug-Seeking Behavior. *Drug discovery today. Disease models*, 5 (4), 207–215.

Cannon, W. B. (1929). Organisation For Physiological Homeostasis. *Physiological Reviews*, 9 (3), 399–431.

Robison, A. J., & Nestler, E. J. (2011). Transcriptional and epigenetic mechanisms of addiction. *Nature reviews. Neuroscience*, 12 (11), 623–637.

Sherman, C. A. R. L. (2007). Impacts of drugs on neurotransmission. *Nida Notes*, 21 (4), 11-15.

Puopolo, M. (2019). The hypothalamic-spinal dopaminergic system: a target for pain modulation. *Neural regeneration research*, 14 (6), 925.

Basbaum, A. I., & Fields, H. L. (1984). Endogenous pain control systems: brainstem spinal pathways and endorphin circuitry. *Annual review of neuroscience*, 7 (1), 309-338.

Landolt, H. P., Meier, V., Burgess, H. J., Finelli, L. A., Cattelin, F., Achermann, P., & Borbély, A. A. (1999). Serotonin-2 receptors and human sleep: effect of a selective antagonist on EEG power spectra. *Neuropsychopharmacology*, 21 (3), 455-466.

Myers, R. D. (1981). Serotonin and thermoregulation: old and new views. *Journal de physiologie*, 77 (2-3), 505-513.

Young, S. N. (2007). How to increase serotonin in the human brain without drugs. *Journal of psychiatry & neuroscience: JPN*, *32* (6), 394.

Barrett, D. (2007). *Waistland: The (R)evolutionary science behind our weight and fitness crisis*. New York: W.W. Norton & Co.

Averill, L. A., Purohit, P., Averill, C. L., Boesl, M. A., Krystal, J. H., & Abdallah, C. G. (2017). Glutamate dysregulation and glutamatergic therapeutics for PTSD: Evidence from human studies. *Neuroscience letters*, *649*, 147-155.

Hyttel, J. (1994). Pharmacological characterization of selective serotonin reuptake inhibitors (SSRIs). *International Clinical Psychopharmacology, 9* (Suppl 1), 19-26.

Sangkuhl, K., Klein, T. E., & Altman, R. B. (2009). Selective serotonin reuptake inhibitors pathway. *Pharmacogenetics and genomics*, 19 (11), 907–909.

Kanherkar, R. R., Getachew, B., Ben-Sheetrit, J., Varma, S., Heinbockel, T., Tizabi, Y., & Csoka, A. B. (2018). The effect of citalopram on genome-wide DNA methylation of human cells. *International journal of genomics*, *2018*.

George, O., Le Moal, M., & Koob, G. F. (2012). Allostasis and addiction: role of the dopamine and corticotropin-releasing factor systems. *Physiology & behavior*, *106* (1), 58–64.

Schulkin, J. (2011). Social allostasis: anticipatory regulation of the internal milieu. *Frontiers in evolutionary neuroscience*, *2*, 111.

Archer, T., Oscar-Berman, M., Blum, K., & Gold, M. S. (2013). Epigenetic modulation of mood disorders. *Journal of genetic syndrome & gene therapy*, *4* (120).

Maze, I., & Nestler, E. J. (2011). The epigenetic landscape of addiction. *Annals of the New York Academy of Sciences*, *1216*, 99–113.

Garrison, G. D., & Dugan, S. E. (2009). Varenicline: a first-line treatment option for smoking cessation. *Clinical therapeutics*, 31 (3), 463-491.

Maloku, E., Kadriu, B., Zhubi, A., Dong, E., Pibiri, F., Satta, R., & Guidotti, A. (2011). Selective α4β2 nicotinic acetylcholine receptor agonists target epigenetic mechanisms in cortical GABAergic neurons. *Neuropsychopharmacology: official publication of the American College of Neuropsychopharmacology*, 36 (7), 1366–1374.

Koob, G. F., Kenneth Lloyd, G., & Mason, B. J. (2009). Development of pharmacotherapies for drug addiction: a Rosetta stone approach. *Nature reviews. Drug discovery*, 8 (6), 500–515.

Thomas, G., Lucas, P., Capler, N. R., Tupper, K. W., & Martin, G. (2013). Ayahuasca-assisted therapy for addiction: results from a preliminary observational study in Canada. *Curr Drug Abuse Rev,* 6 (1), 30-42.

Gasser, P., Holstein, D., Michel, Y., Doblin, R., Yazar-Klosinski, B., Passie, T., & Brenneisen, R. (2014). Safety and efficacy of lysergic acid diethylamide-assisted psychotherapy for anxiety associated with life-threatening diseases. *The Journal of nervous and mental disease,* 202 (7), 513.

Mash, D. C., Duque, L., Page, B., & Allen-Ferdinand, K. (2018). Ibogaine Detoxification Transitions Opioid and Cocaine Abusers Between Dependence and Abstinence: Clinical Observations and Treatment Outcomes. *Frontiers in pharmacology,* 9, 529.

Garcia-Romeu, A., Kersgaard, B., & Addy, P. H. (2016*). Clinical applications of hallucinogens: A review. Experimental and clinical psychopharmacology,* 24 (4), 229–268.

Sessa, B. (2018). Why MDMA therapy for alcohol use disorder? And why now?. *Neuropharmacology*, *142*, 83-88. Riedlinger, T. J., & Riedlinger, J. E. (1994). Psychedelic and entactogenic drugs in the treatment of depression. *Journal of psychoactive drugs*, *26* (1), 41-55.

Ferguson J. M. (2001). SSRI Antidepressant Medications: Adverse Effects and Tolerability. *Primary care companion to the Journal of clinical psychiatry*, 3 (1), 22–27.

Cui, Q., Robinson, L., Elston, D., Smaill, F., Cohen, J., Quan, C., ... & Smieja, M. (2012). Safety and tolerability of varenicline tartrate (Champix®/Chantix®) for smoking cessation in HIV-infected subjects: a pilot open-label study. *AIDS patient care and STDs*, *26* (1), 12-19.

Ruan, H. B., & Crawford, P. A. (2018). Ketone bodies as epigenetic modifiers. *Current Opinion in Clinical Nutrition & Metabolic Care*, *21* (4), 260-266.

Cabrera-Mulero, A., Tinahones, A., Bandera, B., Moreno-Indias, I., Macías-González, M., & Tinahones, F. J. (2019). Keto microbiota: a powerful contributor to host disease recovery. *Reviews in Endocrine and Metabolic Disorders*, *20* (4), 415-425.

Landgrave-Gómez, J., Mercado-Gómez, O., & Guevara-Guzmán, R. (2015). Epigenetic mechanisms in neurological and neurodegenerative diseases. *Frontiers in cellular neuroscience*, 9, 58.

Ketosis

Wheless, J. W. (2008). History of the ketogenic diet. *Epilepsia*, *49* (s8), 3–5.

Fredricks, R. (2013). *Fasting: An exceptional human experience*. Bloomington, IN: AuthorHouse.

Kossoff, E. (2011). *Ketogenic diets: Treatments for epilepsy and other disorders*. New York: Demos Health.

Dashti, H. M., Mathew, T. C., Hussein, T., Asfar, S. K., Behbahani, A., Khoursheed, M. A., Al-Zaid, N. S. (2004). Long-term effects of a ketogenic diet in obese patients. *Experimental and clinical cardiology*, 9 (3), 200–205.

Yancy, W. S., Jr, Foy, M., Chalecki, A. M., Vernon, M. C., & Westman, E. C. (2005). A low-carbohydrate, ketogenic diet to treat type 2 diabetes. *Nutrition & metabolism*, *2*, 34.

Bostock, E. C., Kirkby, K. C., & Taylor, B. V. (2017). The Current Status of the Ketogenic Diet in Psychiatry. *Frontiers in psychiatry*, 8, 43.

Martinez, L. A., Lees, M. E., Ruskin, D. N., & Masino, S. A. (2019). A ketogenic diet diminishes behavioral responses to cocaine in young adult male and female rats. *Neuropharmacology*, 149, 27-34.

Dencker, D., Molander, A., Thomsen, M., Schlumberger, C., Wortwein, G., Weikop, P., ... & Fink-Jensen, A. (2018). Ketogenic diet suppresses alcohol withdrawal syndrome in rats. *Alcoholism: Clinical and Experimental Research,* 42 (2), 270-277.

Castro, A. I., Gomez-Arbelaez, D., Crujeiras, A. B., Granero, R., Aguera, Z., Jimenez-Murcia, S., ... Casanueva, F. F. (2018). Effect of A Very Low-Calorie Ketogenic Diet on Food and Alcohol Cravings, Physical and Sexual Activity, Sleep Disturbances, and Quality of Life in Obese Patients. *Nutrients*, 10 (10), 1348.

D'Andrea Meira, I., Romão, T. T., Pires do Prado, H. J., Krüger, L. T., Pires, M., & da Conceição, P. O. (2019). Ketogenic Diet and Epilepsy: What We Know So Far. *Frontiers in neuroscience*, 13, 5.

Palmer, C. M., Gilbert-Jaramillo, J., & Westman, E. C. (2019). The ketogenic diet and remission of psychotic symptoms in schizophrenia: Two case studies. *Schizophrenia research*, 208, 439.

Kraft, B. D., & Westman, E. C. (2009). Schizophrenia, gluten, and low-carbohydrate, ketogenic diets: a case report and review of the literature. *Nutrition & Metabolism*, 6 (1), 10.

Allen, B. G., Bhatia, S. K., Anderson, C. M., Eichenberger-Gilmore, J. M., Sibenaller, Z. A., Mapuskar, K. A., Fath, M. A. (2014). Ketogenic diets as an adjuvant cancer therapy: History and potential mechanism. *Redox Biology*, 2, 963–970.

Weber, D. D., Aminzadeh-Gohari, S., Tulipan, J., Catalano, L., Feichtinger, R. G., & Kofler, B. (2020). Ketogenic diet in the treatment of cancer—where do we stand?. *Molecular metabolism*, *33*, 102-121.

Fredricks, R. (2013). *Fasting: An exceptional human experience*. Bloomington, IN: AuthorHouse.

Laffel, L. (1999), Ketone bodies: a review of physiology, pathophysiology and application of monitoring to diabetes. *Diabetes Metab. Res. Rev.,* 15: 412-426.

Dhillon, K. K., & Gupta, S. (2018). *Biochemistry, Ketogenesis.* Berg, J. M., Tymoczko, J. L., & Stryer, L. (2002). The citric acid cycle. *Biochemistry*, 465-87.

Vandenberghe, C., St-Pierre, V., Courchesne-Loyer, A., Hennebelle, M., Castellano, C. A., & Cunnane, S. C. (2016). Caffeine intake increases plasma ketones: an acute metabolic study in humans. *Canadian journal of physiology and pharmacology*, 95 (4), 455-458.

Stubbs, B. J., Cox, P. J., Evans, R. D., Santer, P., Miller, J. J., Faull, O. K., ... & Clarke, K. (2017). On the metabolism of exogenous ketones in humans. *Frontiers in physiology*, 8, 848.

Wilson, J., & Lowery, R. (2017). *The Ketogenic Bible: The Authoritative Guide to Ketosis*. Simon and Schuster.

Ward, C. (2019). *Ketone body metabolism - Metabolism and hormones - Diapedia, The Living Textbook of Diabetes.* Retrieved from https://www.Diapdiaorg/51040851169 /rev/29

Rui, L. (2011). Energy metabolism in the liver. *Comprehensive physiology*, 4 (1), 177-197.

Johnson, T. A., Jinnah, H. A., & Kamatani, N. (2019). Shortage of cellular ATP as a cause of diseases and strategies to enhance ATP. *Frontiers in pharmacology*, *10*, 98.

Dean, P., Hirt, R. P., & Embley, T. M. (2016). Microsporidia: Why Make Nucleotides if You Can Steal Them?. *PLoS pathogens*, *12* (11), e1005870.

Dunn, J., & Grider, M. H. (2020). Physiology, Adenosine Triphosphate (ATP).

Asprey, D. (2015). *Bulletproof: The cookbook: lose up to a pound a day, increase your energy, and end food cravings for good :125 recipes to kick ass*. New York: Rodale.

Stubbs, B. J., Cox, P. J., Evans, R. D., Santer, P., Miller, J. J., Faull, O. K., ... & Clarke, K. (2017). On the metabolism of exogenous ketones in humans. *Frontiers in physiology,* 8, 848.

Kesl, S. L., Poff, A. M., Ward, N. P., Fiorelli, T. N., Ari, C., Van Putten, A. J., ... & D'Agostino, D. P. (2016). Effects of exogenous ketone supplementation on blood ketone, glucose, triglyceride, and lipoprotein levels in Sprague-Dawley rats. *Nutrition & metabolism,* 13 (1), 9.

Examine.com. (2019, January 25). *Rhodiola Rosea*. Retrieved from https://examine.com/supplements/rhodiola-rosea.

Mattioli, L., & Perfumi, M. (2007). Rhodiola rosea L. extract reduces stress-and CRF-induced anorexia in rats. *Journal of Psychopharmacology, 21* (7), 742-750.

Darbinyan, V., Aslanyan, G., Amroyan, E., Gabrielyan, E., Malmström, C., & Panossian, A. (2007). Clinical trial of Rhodiola rosea L. extract SHR-5 in the treatment of mild to moderate depression. *Nordic journal of psychiatry, 61* (5), 343-348.

Cifani, C., Di B, M. V. M., Vitale, G., Ruggieri, V., Ciccocioppo, R., & Massi, M. (2010). Effect of salidroside, active principle of Rhodiola rosea extract, on binge eating. *Physiology & behavior*, *101* (5), 555-562.

Kasper, S., & Dienel, A. (2017). Multicenter, open-label, exploratory clinical trial with *Rhodiola rosea* extract in patients suffering from burnout symptoms. *Neuropsychiatric disease and treatment*, *13*, 889–898.

Konstantinos, F., & Heun, R. (2020). The effects of Rhodiola Rosea supplementation on depression, anxiety and mood–A Systematic Review. *Global Psychiatry*, *3* (1), 72-82.

Linde, K., Berner, M., Egger, M., & Mulrow, C. (2005). St John's wort for depression: meta-analysis of randomised controlled trials. *The British Journal of Psychiatry*, *186* (2), 99-107.

Vandenberghe, C., St-Pierre, V., Pierotti, T., Fortier, M., Castellano, C. A., & Cunnane, S. C. (2017). Tricaprylin alone increases plasma Ketone response more than coconut oil or other medium-chain triglycerides: an acute crossover study in healthy adults. *Current developments in nutrition*, 1 (4), e000257.

Zarnowski, T., Tulidowicz-Bielak, M., Kosior-Jarecka, E., Zarnowska, I., A Turski, W., & Gasior, M. (2012). A ketogenic diet may offer neuroprotection in glaucoma and mitochondrial diseases of the optic nerve. *Medical hypothesis, discovery & innovation ophthalmology journal*, 1 (3), 45–49.

Harun-Or-Rashid, M., Pappenhagen, N., Palmer, P. G., Smith, M. A., Gevorgyan, V., Wilson, G. N., Crish, S. D., Inman, D. M. (2018). Structural and Functional Rescue of Chronic Metabolically Stressed Optic Nerves through Respiration. *The Journal of*

neuroscience: *the official journal of the Society for*
Neuroscience, 38 (22), 5122-5139.

D'Andrea Meira, I., Romão, T. T., Pires do Prado, H. J., Krüger, L.
T., Pires, M., & da Conceição, P. O. (2019). Ketogenic Diet and
Epilepsy: What We Know So Far. *Frontiers in neuroscience*, 13, 5.

Gupta, L., Khandelwal, D., Kalra, S., Gupta, P., Dutta, D., &
Aggarwal, S. (2017). Ketogenic diet in endocrine disorders:
Current perspectives. *Journal of postgraduate medicine*,
63 (4), 242–251.

Strandwitz P. (2018). Neurotransmitter modulation by the gut
microbiota. *Brain research*, 1693 (Pt B), 128–133.

Chearskul, S., Delbridge, E., Shulkes, A., Proietto, J., & Kriketos, A.
(2008). Effect of weight loss and ketosis on postprandial
cholecystokinin and free fatty acid concentrations. *The American
journal of clinical nutrition*, 87 (5), 1238-1246.

Miller I. (2018). The gut-brain axis: historical reflections.
Microbial ecology in health and disease, 29 (1), 1542921.

Mazzoli, R., & Pessione, E. (2016). The Neuro-endocrinological
Role of Microbial Glutamate and GABA Signaling. *Frontiers in
microbiology*, 7, 1934.

Samardzic, J., Jadzic, D., Hencic, B., Jancic, J., & Strac, D. S. (2018).
Introductory Chapter: GABA/Glutamate Balance: A Key for
Normal Brain Functioning. GABA And Glutamate: *New
Developments In Neurotransmission Research*, 1.

Kalivas, P. W. (2009). The glutamate homeostasis hypothesis of
addiction. *Nature reviews neuroscience*, 10 (8), 561.

Powledge, T. M. (1999). Addiction and the brain: The dopamine pathway is helping researchers find their way through the addiction maze. *Bioscience*, 49 (7), 513-519.

Avena, N. M., Rada, P., & Hoebel, B. G. (2009). Sugar and fat bingeing have notable differences in addictive-like behavior. *The Journal of nutrition*, *139* (3), 623–628.

Lustig, R. H. (2018). *The hacking of the American mind: The science behind the corporate takeover of our bodies and brains.* New York: Avery, an imprint of Penguin Random House.

Blum, K., Werner, T., Carnes, S., Carnes, P., Bowirrat, A., Giordano, J., … Gold, M. (2012). Sex, drugs, and rock 'n' roll: hypothesizing common mesolimbic activation as a function of reward gene polymorphisms. *Journal of psychoactive drugs*, *44* (1), 38–55.

Bozarth, M. A., & Wise, R. A. (1981). Heroin reward is dependent on a dopaminergic substrate. *Life sciences*, *29* (18), 1881-1886.

Gass, J. T., & Olive, M. F. (2008). Glutamatergic substrates of drug addiction and alcoholism. *Biochemical pharmacology*, 75 (1), 218–265.

Averill, L. A., Purohit, P., Averill, C. L., Boesl, M. A., Krystal, J. H., & Abdallah, C. G. (2017). Glutamate dysregulation and glutamatergic therapeutics for PTSD: Evidence from human studies. *Neuroscience letters*, *649*, 147-155.

Khoury, L., Tang, Y. L., Bradley, B., Cubells, J. F., & Ressler, K. J. (2010). Substance use, childhood traumatic experience, and posttraumatic stress disorder in an urban civilian population. *Depression and Anxiety*, *27* (12), 1077-1086.

Cho C. H. (2013). New mechanism for glutamate hypothesis in epilepsy. *Frontiers in cellular neuroscience*, 7, 127.

Sanacora, G., Treccani, G., & Popoli, M. (2012). Towards a glutamate hypothesis of depression: an emerging frontier of neuropsychopharmacology for mood disorders. *Neuropharmacology*, 62 (1), 63–77.

Pittenger, C., Bloch, M. H., & Williams, K. (2011). Glutamate abnormalities in obsessive compulsive disorder: neurobiology, pathophysiology, and treatment. *Pharmacology & therapeutics*, 132 (3), 314–332.

Benussi, A., Alberici, A., Buratti, E., Ghidoni, R., Gardoni, F., Di Luca, M., ... & Borroni, B. (2019). Toward a Glutamate Hypothesis of Frontotemporal Dementia. *Frontiers in neuroscience*, 13.

Moghaddam, B., & Javitt, D. (2012). From revolution to evolution: the glutamate hypothesis of schizophrenia and its implication for treatment. *Neuropsychopharmacology: official publication of the American College of Neuropsychopharmacology*, 37 (1), 4–15.

Shinohe, A., Hashimoto, K., Nakamura, K., Tsujii, M., Iwata, Y., Tsuchiya, K. J., ... & Matsuzaki, H. (2006). Increased serum levels of glutamate in adult patients with autism. *Progress in Neuro-Psychopharmacology and Biological Psychiatry*, 30 (8), 1472-1477.

Hartman, A. L., Gasior, M., Vining, E. P., & Rogawski, M. A. (2007). The neuropharmacology of the ketogenic diet. *Pediatric neurology*, 36 (5), 281–292.

Yudkoff, M., Daikhin, Y., Horyn, O., Nissim, I., & Nissim, I. (2008). Ketosis and brain handling of glutamate, glutamine, and GABA. *Epilepsia*, 49 Suppl 8 (Suppl 8), 73–75.

Petroff, O. A. (2002). Book review: GABA and glutamate in the human brain. *The Neuroscientist*, 8 (6), 562-573.

Nance, E. A. (2018). Ketogenic bugs as epilepsy drugs. *Science Translational Medicine*, *10* (446), eaau0471.

What Ketosis and a Ketogenic diet can treat, prevent or improve.

Scientific evidence

Paoli, A., Grimaldi, K., Toniolo, L., Canato, M., Bianco, A., & Fratter, A. (2012). Nutrition and acne: therapeutic potential of ketogenic diets. *Skin pharmacology and physiology*, 25 (3), 111-117.

Martinez, L. A., Lees, M. E., Ruskin, D. N., & Masino, S. A. (2019). A ketogenic diet diminishes behavioral responses to cocaine in young adult male and female rats. *Neuropharmacology*, 149, 27-34.

Castro, A. I., Gomez-Arbelaez, D., Crujeiras, A. B., Granero, R., Aguera, Z., Jimenez-Murcia, S., ... Casanueva, F. F. (2018). Effect of A Very Low-Calorie Ketogenic Diet on Food and Alcohol Cravings, Physical and Sexual Activity, Sleep Disturbances, and Quality of Life in Obese Patients. *Nutrients*, 10 (10), 1348.

Carmen, M., Safer, D. L., Saslow, L. R., Kalayjian, T., Mason, A. E., Westman, E. C., & Dalai, S. S. (2020). Treating binge eating and food addiction symptoms with low-carbohydrate Ketogenic diets: a case series. *Journal of eating disorders*, 8 (1), 1-7.

Zilberter, T., & Zilberter, Y. (2018). Ketogenic ratio determines metabolic effects of macronutrients and prevents interpretive bias. *Frontiers in nutrition*, 5, 75.

Jurecka, A., Zikanova, M., Kmoch, S., & Tylki-Szymańska, A. (2015). Adenylosuccinate lyase deficiency. *Journal of inherited metabolic disease*, 38 (2), 231–242.

Roberts, M. N., Wallace, M. A., Tomilov, A. A., Zhou, Z., Marcotte, G. R., Tran, D., ... Lopez-Dominguez, J. A. (2017). A Ketogenic Diet Extends Longevity and Healthspan in Adult Mice. *Cell metabolism*, 26 (3), 539–546.e5.

Włodarek D. (2019). Role of Ketogenic Diets in Neurodegenerative Diseases (Alzheimer's Disease and Parkinson's Disease). *Nutrients,* 11 (1), 169.

Zhao, Z., Lange, D. J., Voustianiouk, A., MacGrogan, D., Ho, L., Suh, J., ... & Pasinetti, G. M. (2006). A ketogenic diet as a potential novel therapeutic intervention in amyotrophic lateral sclerosis. *BMC neuroscience,* 7 (1), 29.

Grocott, O. R., Herrington, K. S., Pfeifer, H. H., Thiele, E. A., & Thibert, R. L. (2017). Low glycemic index treatment for seizure control in Angelman syndrome: A case series from the Center for Dietary Therapy of Epilepsy at the Massachusetts General Hospital. *Epilepsy & Behavior*, 68, 45-50.

Bostock, E. C. S., Kirkby, K. C., & Taylor, B. V. M. (2017). The Current Status of the Ketogenic Diet in Psychiatry. *Frontiers in Psychiatry*, 8, 43.

Gibson, A. A., Seimon, R. V., Lee, C. M., Ayre, J., Franklin, J., Markovic, T. P., ... & Sainsbury, A. (2015). Do ketogenic diets really suppress appetite? A systematic review and meta-analysis. *Obesity Reviews,* 16 (1), 64-76.

Scolnick, B., Zupec-Kania, B., Calabrese, L., Aoki, C., & Hildebrandt, T. (2020). Remission from Chronic Anorexia Nervosa With Ketogenic Diet and Ketamine: Case Report. *Frontiers in Psychiatry,* 11, 763.

Scolnick, B. (2017). Ketogenic diet and anorexia nervosa. *Medical Hypotheses*, *109*, 150-152.

Napoli, E., Dueñas, N., & Giulivi, C. (2014). Potential therapeutic use of the ketogenic diet in autism spectrum disorders. *Frontiers in pediatrics*, 2, 69.

Campbell, I. H., & Campbell, H. (2019). Ketosis and bipolar disorder: controlled analytic study of online reports. *BJPsych Open*, 5 (4), e58.

Kosinski, C., & Jornayvaz, F. R. (2017). Effects of Ketogenic Diets on Cardiovascular Risk Factors: Evidence from Animal and Human Studies. *Nutrients*, 9 (5), 517.

McDougall, A., Bayley, M., & Munce, S. E. (2018). The ketogenic diet as a treatment for traumatic brain injury: a scoping review. *Brain injury*, 32 (4), 416-422.

Tan-Shalaby J. (2017). Ketogenic Diets and Cancer: Emerging Evidence. *Federal practitioner: for the health care professionals of the VA, DoD, and PHS,* 34 (Suppl 1), 37S–42S.

Marsh, J., Mukherjee, P., & Seyfried, T. N. (2008). Drug/diet synergy for managing malignant astrocytoma in mice: 2-deoxy-D-glucose and the restricted ketogenic diet. *Nutrition & metabolism,* 5 (1), 33.

Weber, D. D., Aminazdeh-Gohari, S., & Kofler, B. (2018). Ketogenic diet in cancer therapy. *Aging,* 10 (2), 164–165.

Otto, C., Kaemmerer, U., Illert, B., Muehling, B., Pfetzer, N., Wittig, R., ... & Coy, J. F. (2008). Growth of human gastric cancer cells in nude mice is delayed by a ketogenic diet supplemented with omega-3 fatty acids and medium-chain triglycerides. *BMC cancer,* 8 (1), 122.

Zhou, W., Mukherjee, P., Kiebish, M. A., Markis, W. T., Mantis, J. G., & Seyfried, T. N. (2007). The calorically restricted ketogenic diet, an effective alternative therapy for malignant brain cancer. *Nutrition & metabolism*, 4, 5.

Klement R. J. (2014). Restricting carbohydrates to fight head and neck cancer-is this realistic?. *Cancer biology & medicine*, 11 (3), 145–161.

Schwartz, K. A., Noel, M., Nikolai, M., & Chang, H. T. (2018). Investigating the ketogenic diet as treatment for primary aggressive brain cancer: challenges and lessons learned. *Frontiers in nutrition*, 5, 11.

van der Louw, E., Olieman, J. F., van den Bemt, P., Bromberg, J., Oomen-de Hoop, E., Neuteboom, R. F., Catsman-Berrevoets, C. E., & Vincent, A. (2019). Ketogenic diet treatment as adjuvant to standard treatment of glioblastoma multiforme: a feasibility and safety study. *Therapeutic advances in medical oncology*, *11*, 1758835919853958.

Morscher, R. J., Aminzadeh-Gohari, S., Feichtinger, R. G., Mayr, J. A., Lang, R., Neureiter, D., ... Kofler, B. (2015). Inhibition of Neuroblastoma Tumor Growth by Ketogenic Diet and/or Calorie Restriction in a CD1-Nu Mouse Model. *PloS one,* 10 (6), e0129802.

Al-Zaid, N. S., Dashti, H. M., Mathew, T. C., & Juggi, J. S. (2007). Low carbohydrate ketogenic diet enhances cardiac tolerance to global ischaemia. *Acta cardiologica*, 62 (4), 381-389.

Lim, Z., Wong, K., Olson, H. E., Bergin, A. M., Downs, J., & Leonard, H. (2017). Use of the ketogenic diet to manage refractory epilepsy in CDKL 5 disorder: Experience of 100 patients. *Epilepsia,* 58 (8), 1415-1422.

Krikorian, R., Shidler, M. D., Dangelo, K., Couch, S. C., Benoit, S. C., & Clegg, D. J. (2012). Dietary ketosis enhances memory in mild cognitive impairment. *Neurobiology of aging,* 33 (2), 425-e19.

Hernandez, A. R., Hernandez, C. M., Campos, K., Truckenbrod, L., Federico, Q., Moon, B., ... & Burke, S. N. (2018). A ketogenic diet improves cognition and has biochemical effects in prefrontal cortex that are dissociable from hippocampus. *Frontiers in aging neuroscience*, 10.

D'Andrea Meira, I., Romão, T. T., Pires do Prado, H. J., Krüger, L. T., Pires, M., & da Conceição, P. O. (2019). Ketogenic Diet and Epilepsy: What We Know So Far. *Frontiers in neuroscience*, 13, 5.

Tóth, C., Dabóczi, A., Howard, M., Miller, N. J., & Clemens, Z. (2016). Crohn's disease successfully treated with the paleolithic ketogenic diet. *Int. J. Case Rep*. Images, 7, 570-578.

Murphy, P., Likhodii, S., Nylen, K., & Burnham, W. M. (2004). The antidepressant properties of the ketogenic diet. *Biological psychiatry*, 56 (12), 981-983.

El-Mallakh, R. S., & Paskitti, M. E. (2001). The ketogenic diet may have mood-stabilizing properties. *Medical hypotheses*, 57 (6), 724-726.

Yancy, W. S., Jr, Foy, M., Chalecki, A. M., Vernon, M. C., & Westman, E. C. (2005). A low-carbohydrate, ketogenic diet to treat type 2 diabetes. *Nutrition & metabolism*, 2, 34.

Davis, J. J., Fournakis, N., & Ellison, J. (2021). Ketogenic diet for the treatment and prevention of dementia: a review. *Journal of geriatric psychiatry and neurology*, *34* (1), 3-10.

McSwiney, F. T., Wardrop, B., Hyde, P. N., Lafountain, R. A., Volek, J. S., & Doyle, L. (2018). Keto-adaptation enhances exercise performance and body composition responses to training in endurance athletes. *Metabolism*, *81*, 25-34.

Alwahab, U. A., Pantalone, K. M., & Burguera, B. (2018). A ketogenic diet may restore fertility in women with polycystic ovary syndrome: a case series. *AACE Clinical Case Reports,* 4 (5), e427-e431.

Zarnowski, T., Tulidowicz-Bielak, M., Kosior-Jarecka, E., Zarnowska, I., A Turski, W., & Gasior, M. (2012). A ketogenic diet may offer neuroprotection in glaucoma and mitochondrial diseases of the optic nerve. *Medical hypothesis, discovery & innovation ophthalmology journal*, 1 (3), 45–49.

Spalice, A., & Guido, C. A. (2018). Cardiovascular Risks of Ketogenic Diet for Glut-1 Deficiency. *Pediatric neurology briefs*, 32, 8.

Olson, C. A., Vuong, H. E., Yano, J. M., Liang, Q. Y., Nusbaum, D. J., & Hsiao, E. Y. (2018). The gut microbiota mediates the anti-seizure effects of the ketogenic diet. *Cell*, 173 (7), 1728-1741.

Dashti, H. M., Bo-Abbas, Y. Y., Asfar, S. K., Mathew, T. C., Hussein, T., Behbahani, A., ... & Al-Zaid, N. S. (2003). Ketogenic diet modifies the risk factors of heart disease in obese patients. *Nutrition*, *19* (10), 901.

Morrison, S. A., Fazeli, P. L., Gower, B., Younger, J., Willig, A., Sneed, N. M., & Vance, D. E. (2018). The ketogenic diet as a non-pharmacological treatment for HIV-associated neurocognitive disorder: A descriptive analysis. *Journal of psychiatry and behavioral science*, 3, 1014.

Gupta, L., Khandelwal, D., Kalra, S., Gupta, P., Dutta, D., & Aggarwal, S. (2017). Ketogenic diet in endocrine disorders: Current perspectives. *Journal of postgraduate medicine*, 63 (4), 242–251.

Ruskin, D. N., Ross, J. L., Kawamura Jr, M., Ruiz, T. L., Geiger, J. D., & Masino, S. A. (2011). A ketogenic diet delays weight loss and does not impair working memory or motor function in the R6/2 1J mouse model of Huntington's disease. *Physiology & behavior*, 103 (5), 501-507.

Ma, S., & Suzuki, K. (2019). Keto-Adaptation and Endurance Exercise Capacity, Fatigue Recovery, and Exercise-Induced Muscle and Organ Damage Prevention: A Narrative Review. *Sports (Basel, Switzerland)*, *7* (2), 40.

Zajac, A., Poprzecki, S., Maszczyk, A., Czuba, M., Michalczyk, M., & Zydek, G. (2014). The effects of a ketogenic diet on exercise metabolism and physical performance in off-road cyclists. *Nutrients*, 6 (7), 2493–2508.

Pinto, A., Bonucci, A., Maggi, E., Corsi, M., & Businaro, R. (2018). Anti-Oxidant and Anti-Inflammatory Activity of Ketogenic Diet: New Perspectives for Neuroprotection in Alzheimer's Disease. *Antioxidants (Basel, Switzerland)*, 7 (5), 63.

Austin, G. L., Dalton, C. B., Hu, Y., Morris, C. B., Hankins, J., Weinland, S. R., ... Drossman, D. A. (2009). A very low-carbohydrate diet improves symptoms and quality of life in diarrhea-predominant irritable bowel syndrome. *Clinical gastroenterology and hepatology: the official clinical practice journal of the American Gastroenterological Association,* 7 (6), 706–708.e1.

Cardinali, S., Canafoglia, L., Bertoli, S., Franceschetti, S., Lanzi, G., Tagliabue, A., & Veggiotti, P. (2006). A pilot study of a ketogenic diet in patients with Lafora body disease. *Epilepsy research,* 69 (2), 129-134.

Vorgerd, M., & Zange, J. (2007). Treatment of glycogenosys type V (McArdle disease) with creatine and ketogenic diet with clinical scores and with 31P-MRS on working leg muscle. *Acta myologica: myopathies and cardiomyopathies: official journal of the Mediterranean Society of Myology,* 26 (1), 61–63.

SCHNABEL, T. G. (1928). An experience with a ketogenic dietary in migraine. *Annals of Internal Medicine,* 2 (4), 341-347.

Paleologou, E., Ismayilova, N., & Kinali, M. (2017). Use of the Ketogenic Diet to Treat Intractable Epilepsy in Mitochondrial Disorders. *Journal of clinical medicine*, 6 (6), 56.

Brietzke, E., Mansur, R. B., Subramaniapillai, M., Balanzá-Martínez, V., Vinberg, M., González-Pinto, A., ... & McIntyre, R. S. (2018). Ketogenic diet as a metabolic therapy for mood disorders: evidence and developments. *Neuroscience & Biobehavioral Reviews*, 94, 11-16.

Storoni, M., & Plant, G. T. (2015). The Therapeutic Potential of the Ketogenic Diet in Treating Progressive Multiple Sclerosis. *Multiple sclerosis international, 2015*, 681289.

Husain, A. M., Yancy, W. S., Carwile, S. T., Miller, P. P., & Westman, E. C. (2004). Diet therapy for narcolepsy. *Neurology,* 62 (12), 2300-2302.

Schugar, R. C., & Crawford, P. A. (2012). Low-carbohydrate ketogenic diets, glucose homeostasis, and nonalcoholic fatty liver disease. *Current opinion in clinical nutrition and metabolic care*, *15* (4), 374.

Tendler, D., Lin, S., Yancy, W. S., Mavropoulos, J., Sylvestre, P., Rockey, D. C., & Westman, E. C. (2007). The effect of a low-carbohydrate, ketogenic diet on nonalcoholic fatty liver disease: a pilot study. *Digestive diseases and sciences*, *52* (2), 589-593.

Gasior, M., Rogawski, M. A., & Hartman, A. L. (2006). Neuroprotective and disease-modifying effects of the ketogenic diet. *Behavioural pharmacology,* 17 (5-6), 431–439.

Sivaraju, A., Nussbaum, I., Cardoza, C. S., & Mattson, R. H. (2015). Substantial and sustained seizure reduction with ketogenic diet in a patient with Ohtahara syndrome. *Epilepsy & behavior case reports*, 3, 43-45.

Masino, S. A., & Ruskin, D. N. (2013). Ketogenic diets and pain. *Journal of child neurology*, 28 (8), 993–1001.

Swoboda, K. J., Specht, L., Jones, H. R., Shapiro, F., DiMauro, S., & Korson, M. (1997). Infantile phosphofructokinase deficiency with arthrogryposis: clinical benefit of a ketogenic diet. *The Journal of pediatrics,* 131 (6), 932-*934.*

Sofou, K., Dahlin, M., Hallböök, T., Lindefeldt, M., Viggedal, G., & Darin, N. (2017). Ketogenic diet in pyruvate dehydrogenase complex deficiency: short- and long-term outcomes. *Journal of inherited metabolic disease*, 40 (2), 237–245.

Elamin, M., Ruskin, D. N., Masino, S. A., & Sacchetti, P. (2018). Ketogenic Diet Modulates NAD^+-Dependent Enzymes and Reduces DNA Damage in Hippocampus. *Frontiers in cellular neuroscience*, 12, 263.

Liebhaber, G. M., Riemann, E., & Matthias Baumeister, F. A. (2003). Ketogenic diet in Rett syndrome. *Journal of child neurology,* 18 (1), 74-75.

Khanna, S., Jaiswal, K. S., & Gupta, B. (2017). Managing Rheumatoid Arthritis with Dietary Interventions. *Frontiers in nutrition*, 4, 52.

Kraft, B. D., & Westman, E. C. (2009). Schizophrenia, gluten, and low-carbohydrate, ketogenic diets: a case report and review of the literature. *Nutrition & Metabolism*, 6 (1), 10.

Shaafi, S., Mahmoudi, J., Pashapour, A., Farhoudi, M., Sadigh-Eteghad, S., & Akbari, H. (2014). Ketogenic Diet Provides Neuroprotective Effects against Ischemic Stroke Neuronal Damages. *Advanced pharmaceutical bulletin*, 4 (Suppl 2), 479–481.

Bautista, R. E. D. (2003). The use of the ketogenic diet in a patient with subacute sclerosing panencephalitis. *Seizure,* 12 (3), 175–177.

Paoli, A., Rubini, A., Volek, J. S., & Grimaldi, K. A. (2013). Beyond weight loss: a review of the therapeutic uses of very-low-carbohydrate (ketogenic) diets. *European journal of clinical nutrition,* 67 (8), *789.*

Dencker, D., Molander, A., Thomsen, M., Schlumberger, C., Wortwein, G., Weikop, P., ... & Fink-Jensen, A. (2018). Ketogenic diet suppresses alcohol withdrawal syndrome in rats. *Alcoholism: Clinical and Experimental Research*, 42 (2), 270-277.

Anecdotal reports

Gyrlgeorge. (2018, November 22). Keto "cured" my alcoholism! : keto. *Reddit.com*. Retrieved from https://www .reddit.com/r/keto/comments/9z9s9e/keto_cured_my_alcoh olism

AddictChick. (2018, May 4). Keto and recovering drug addicts. *Reddit.com*. Retrieved from https://www.reddit. com/r/keto/comments/8h15hz/keto_and_recovering_drug_a ddicts

Cannavis. (2019, March 23). Is this the cure for depression and anxiety? I think Keto has helped me is a much much bigger way. *Reddit.com*. Retrieved fromhttps://www.reddit. com/r/keto/comments/b4p2hr/is_this_the_cure_for_depress ion_and_anxiety_i

greenbeanjellybean. (2014, December 13). Eating disorders and keto. *Reddit.com*. Retrieved from https://www.reddit .com/r/keto/comments/2p78jj/eating_disorders_and_keto/

Dashund123. (2015, March 31). Binge Eating/Eating disorder cured with Keto. *Reddit.com*. Retrieved from https://www. reddit.com/r/keto/comments/30ys6z/binge_eatingeating _disorder_cured_with_keto/

icegurl. (2016, July 28). Anyone battling bulimia? *Reddit.com*. Retrieved from https://www.reddit.com/r/keto/comments /4uzm4h/anyone_battling_bulimia/

yellowumbrella. (2020, December 26). The Keto Diet Helped Me Overcome Fast Food Addiction. *Reddit.com*. Retrieved from https://www.reddit.com/r/HealthyZapper/comments/ kkmq46/the_keto_diet_helped_me_overcome_fast_food/

Natalicious-Keto. (2019, September 25). 54F, 5'10" I'm Down 110 lbs in Under 18 Months and Feeling Fabulous AF!!!. *Reddit.com*. Retrieved from https://www.reddit.com/r/Keto/comments/d959j4/54f_510_im_down_110_lbs_in_under_18_months_and

tcookie88. (2019, August 02). Keto has really helped my arthritis. *Reddit.com*. Retrieved from https://www.reddit.com/r/keto/comments/cl492a/keto_has_really_helped_my_arthritis

Slithybooks. (2018, September 28). Bipolar & Keto: A Story. *Reddit.com*. Retrieved from https://www.reddit.com/r/keto/comments/9jqf2h/bipolar_keto_a_story

NateTay. (2019, October 28). KETO - Blood Pressure - Before and After. *Reddit.com*. Retrieved from https://www.reddit.com/r/keto/comments/do2qub/keto_blood_pressure_before_and_after

mfk96. (2019, October 21). I have been on keto for 30 months, omad for 12 months, and 90% carnivore for 6 months. Have lost 55Kg, no floppy skin, rejuvenated 20 years, my white hair turned black again, much better breathing, much better intelectual capacity, and I have improvements on my health that I can't even describe. *Reddit.com*. Retrieved from https://www.reddit.com/r/keto/comments/dl6p10/i_have_been_on_keto_for_30_months_omad_for_12

TheMikeFly. (2018, November 29). Non-Alcoholic Fatty Liver Disease and Keto - a 1 year journey *SPOILER* I got it under control. *Reddit.com*. Retrieved from https://www.reddit.com/r/keto/comments/a1d4jl/nonalcoholic_fatty_liver_disease_and_keto_a_1/

NotoriousBRT. (2019, January 15). Keto energy boost? . *Reddit.com*. Retrieved from https://www.reddit.com/ r/keto/comments/ag5wuy/keto_energy_boost

gyozaz64. (2019, June 04). Keto and Concentration. *Reddit.com*. Retrieved from https://www.reddit.com /r/keto/comments/bwpbbo/keto_and_concentration

i_heart_pigeons. (2019, March 07). Keto fixed my stomach! Anyone know the science behind it?. *Reddit.com*. Retrieved from https://www.reddit.com/r/keto/comments/ay8roy /keto_fixed_my_stomach_anyone_know_the_science

JenRf. (2019, March 07). *Hormonal imbalances, depression & Keto. I could not be more grateful!!!! Reddit.com*. Retrieved from https://www.reddit.com/r/keto/comments/9bc299 /hormonal_imbalances_depression_keto_i_could_not

_ICE_COLD_WATER_5. (2019, May 08). So Keto is something else. *Reddit.com*. Retrieved fromhttps://www.reddit.com /r/keto/comments/bm9tw2/so_keto_is_something_else

FountainPenandInk. (2019, October 12). [NSV] My Vision Improved. *Reddit.com*. Retrieved from https://www.reddit. com/r/keto/comment/dgybi3/nsv_my_vision_improved

ketogal1990. (2017, September 12). Reduced inflammation on keto? *Reddit.com*. Retrieved from https://www.reddit. com/r/keto/comments/6zjn3r/reduced_inflammation_on_ke to

crossmyheartxx. (2013, October 25). My IBS symptoms were completely reversed when I embarked on the ketogenic journey.*Reddit.com*. Retrieved from https://www.reddit.

com/r/keto/comments/1p71lw/my_ibs_symptoms_were_co
mpletely_reversed_when_i

hash_code_u. (2021, January 12). keto for brain [focus &
mood]. need anecdotal reference. *Reddit.com*. Retrieved
from https://www.reddit.com/r/keto/comments/kvw4m0
/keto_for_brain_focus_mood_need_anecdotal_reference/

ElGrandeQues0. (2021, February 18). Male, 30 years old and
one month Keto - No longer Obese! *Reddit.com*. Retrieved
from https://www.reddit.com/r/keto/comments/lmu4tm
/male_30_years_old_and_one_month_keto_no_longer/

Decent_Cook_2707. (2021, February 18). Former obese men
whom reached their ideal body weight keto, and then
reached 15% body fat (or lower) through a recomp - how
exactly did you succeed doing the recomp? *Reddit.com*.
Retrieved from https://www.reddit.com/r/keto/comments
/lk9bsq/fomer_obese_men_whom_reached_their_ideal_bod
y/

Becca941. (2019, July 13). Trying keto for PTSD, 3 days in and
hopeful 😊 *Reddit.com*. Retrieved from https://www.reddit.
com/r/Keto/comments/ccnh07/trying_keto_for_ptsd_3_days
_in_and_hopeful/

Keto Savage. (2019, August 6). BRANDON CLARK ON KETO
FOR PTSD AND TRAINING EXCLUSIVELY WITH RESISTANCE
BANDS AND BODYWEIGHT! *KETO SAVAGE PRIMAL
PERFORMANCE*. Retrieved from https://ketosavage.com
/brandon-clark-on-keto-for-ptsd-and-training-exclusively-
with-resistance-bands-and-bodyweight/

PaleFactor. (2018, December 11). Keto for Recovery from Schizophrenia. *Reddit.com*. Retrieved from https://www.reddit.com/r/keto/comments/a52z4g/keto_for_recovery_from_schizophrenia

scheto. (2013, May 02). Keto and schizophrenia - my story. *Reddit.com*. Retrievedfromhttps://www.reddit.com/r/keto/comments/1djuha/keto_and_schizophrenia_my_story/

thehorrorr. (2016, May 06). [NSV] I have type 2 diabetes. This chart shows my blood sugar levels after starting a keto diet. It works!. *Reddit.com.* Retrieved from https://www.reddit.com/r/keto/comments/4i4wmu/nsv_i_have_type_2_diabetes_this_chart_shows_my

slimyagent. (2019, March 03). The only love that doesn't need a prenup: Keto changed my life (despite my own best efforts). *Reddit.com*. Retrieved from https://www.reddit.com/r/keto/comments/awvj8k/the_only_love_that_doesnt_need_a_prenup_keto

the_reverence. (2020, May 17). Keto and Ulcerative Colitis, looking for timelines/testimonials. *Reddit.com*. Retrieved from https://www.reddit.com/r/keto/comments/gl9cnt/keto_and_ulcerative_colitis_looking_for/

Zealous_Zebras. (2021, January 20). Going on week 2: alcohol abstinent with 6 lb weight gain. *Reddit.com*. Retrieved from https://www.reddit.com/r/keto/comments/l1kb6z/going_on_week_2_alcohol_abstinent_with_6_lb/

Coconut Ketosis

Norgren, J., Sindi, S., Sandebring-Matton, A., Kåreholt, I., Daniilidou, M., Akenine, U., ... & Kivipelto, M. (2020). Ketosis After Intake of Coconut Oil and Caprylic Acid—With and Without Glucose: A Cross-Over Study in Healthy Older Adults. *Frontiers in nutrition, 7*, 40.

Prasad, S., Tyagi, A. K., & Aggarwal, B. B. (2014). Recent developments in delivery, bioavailability, absorption and metabolism of curcumin: the golden pigment from golden spice. *Cancer research and treatment: official journal of Korean Cancer Association*, *46* (1), 2–18.

Srinivasan, K. (2007). Black pepper and its pungent principle-piperine: a review of diverse physiological effects. *Critical reviews in food science and nutrition*, *47* (8), 735-748.

McCarty, M. F., DiNicolantonio, J. J., & O'Keefe, J. H. (2015). Capsaicin may have important potential for promoting vascular and metabolic health. *Open heart*, *2* (1), e000262.

Clegg, M. E., Golsorkhi, M., & Henry, C. J. (2013). Combined medium-chain triglyceride and chilli feeding increases diet-induced thermogenesis in normal-weight humans. European journal of nutrition, 52 (6), 1579-1585.

Charry, J. M. (2018). *Air Ions: Physical and Biological Aspects.* Boca Raton, FL: CRC Press.

Perez, V., Alexander, D. D., & Bailey, W. H. (2013). Air ions and mood outcomes: a review and meta analysis. BMC psychiatry, 13, 29.

Macomber, S. (2013). *Our electric emotions: What actually causes mental/emotional illnesses? is there a way to reverse them?*. Bloomington, Ind.: Xlibris.

Russell, W. (1974). *The Universal One.* Swannanoa, Waynesboro, Virginia: University of Science and Philosophy.

Russell, W. (1994). *The Secret of Light.* Swannanoa, Waynesboro, Virginia: University of Science and Philosophy.

Smith, J. J. (2015). *Lose weight without dieting or working out: Discover secrets to a slimmer, sexier, and healthier you.* New York: Atria Books.

Chia, M., Dao, J. (2017). The Eight Immortal Healers: Taoist Wisdom for Radiant Health. United States: Inner Traditions/Bear.

Gračanin, A., Bylsma, L. M., & Vingerhoets, A. J. (2014). Is crying a self-soothing behavior?. *Frontiers in psychology*, 5, 502.

Kemp, D., & Daly, P. (2016). *The Ketogenic Kitchen: Low carb. High fat. Extraordinary health.* Dublin: Gill & Macmillan.

Harvey, C., Schofield, G. M., & Williden, M. (2018). The use of nutritional supplements to induce ketosis and reduce symptoms associated with keto-induction: a narrative review. *PeerJ*, 6, e4488.

Mancinelli, K. (2014). *The Ketogenic Diet: A Scientifically Proven Approach to Fast, Healthy Weight Loss.* Berkeley, CA: Ulysses

Spritzler, F., & Scher, B. (2019, May 13). Our comprehensive guide to salt. *Diet Doctor*. Retrieved from https://www.dietdoctor.com/low-carb/salt-guide#on-keto.

McDonald, L., & McDonald, L. (1998). *The ketogenic diet: A complete guide for the dieter and practitioner*. Austin, TX: The Author.

Rodin, J. (1985). Insulin levels, hunger, and food intake: an example of feedback loops in body weight regulation. *Health Psychology*, 4 (1), 1.

Cronometer (2019). *Cronometer: Track Your Nutrition, Fitness, & Health Data, Log your Diet, Exercise, Biometrics and Notes.* Retrieved from https://cronometer.com/

Kalivas, P. W. (2009). The glutamate homeostasis hypothesis of addiction. *Nature reviews neuroscience*, 10 (8), 561.

Cabrera-Mulero, A., Tinahones, A., Bandera, B., Moreno-Indias, I., Macías-González, M., & Tinahones, F. J. (2019). Keto microbiota: a powerful contributor to host disease recovery. *Reviews in Endocrine and Metabolic Disorders*, *20* (4), 415-425.

Mazzoli, R., & Pessione, E. (2016). The Neuro-endocrinological Role of Microbial Glutamate and GABA Signaling. *Frontiers in microbiology*, *7*, 1934.

Abrams, R., Abrams, V. (2019). *Keto Diet For Dummies*. United Kingdom: Wiley.

The Treatment of Obesity. (1979). *United States:* University Park Press.

Pietrzykowski, A. Z., & Treistman, S. N. (2008). The molecular basis of tolerance. *Alcohol research & health: the journal of the National Institute on Alcohol Abuse and Alcoholism*, *31* (4), 298–309.

Sybertz, A. (2020). *The OMAD Diet: Intermittent Fasting with One Meal a Day to Burn Fat and Lose Weight.* United States: Ulysses Press.

Wilkinsen, M. (2019). *The Keto OMAD Diet: How to Combine the Ketogenic Diet with the One Meal A Day Intermittent Fasting Diet to Maximize Your Weight Loss. (n.p.):* INDEPENDENTLY PUBLISHED.

MacDowell, L. (2018). *Vegan Keto*. United States: Victory Belt Publishing.

Fredricks, R. (2012). *Fasting: an Exceptional Human Experience*. United States: AuthorHouse.

Gallagher, E. V, & Willsky-Ciollo, L. (2021*). New Religions: Emerging Faiths and Religious Cultures in the Modern World [2 volumes]*. ABC-CLIO.

Kemp, D., & Daly, P. (2016). *The Ketogenic Kitchen: Low carb. High fat. Extraordinary health*. Dublin: Gill & Macmillan.

Saylor, C. P. (2006). *Weight loss, exercise and health research*. New York: Nova Science Publishers.

Moore, J., Rushin, H. (2019). *Keto Clarity Cookbook: Your Definitive Guide to Cooking Low-Carb, High-Fat Meals*. United States: Victory Belt Publishing.

Eenfeldt, A. (2021, March 05). How low carb is keto?. *Diet Doctor*. Retrieved fromhttps://www.dietdoctor.com /low-carb/keto/how-low-carb-is-keto

Carandang, E. V. (2008). Health benefits of virgin coconut oil. *INDIAN COCONUT JOURNAL-COCHIN-*, *38* (9), 8

Dhillon, K. K., & Gupta, S. (2018). *Biochemistry, Ketogenesis.*

Zuckerman, J. M., & Assimos, D. G. (2009). Hypocitraturia: pathophysiology and medical management. *Reviews in urology*, *11* (3), 134–144.

Penniston, K. L., Nakada, S. Y., Holmes, R. P., & Assimos, D. G. (2008). Quantitative assessment of citric acid in lemon juice, lime juice, and commercially-available fruit juice products. *Journal of endourology,* 22 (3), 567–570.

Paoli, A., Bosco, G., Camporesi, E. M., & Mangar, D. (2015). Ketosis, ketogenic diet and food intake control: a complex relationship. *Frontiers in psychology,* 6, 27.

Graham, D. N. (2010). *The 80/10/10 diet: Balancing your health, your weight, and your life one luscious bite at a time.* Key Largo, Fla: FoodnSport Press.

Cousens, G. (2000). *Conscious eating.* Berkeley, Calif: North Atlantic Books.

Cousens, G., & Tree of Life Café. (2003). *Rainbow green live-food cuisine*. Berkeley, Calif: North Atlantic Books.

Lee, M. (2017). *Vegan Keto: 70 Healthy & Delicious Low-carb Recipes*. Norway: Pine Peak Publishing.

Nwozo, A. (2019). *The Raw Ketogenic Diet: The Raw Keto Approach to Great Health, Amazing Energy and Permanent Weight Loss Including a 14 day Meal Plan With Net Carbs under 25 g per day!* [Kindle Edition].

Stone, G., Campbell, T. C., & Esselstyn, C. B. (2012). *Forks over knives: The plant-based way to health*. Camberwell, Vic: Penguin Group.

LaBar, D. (2017). *Simple. Natural. Healing: A common sense approach to total health transformation*. New York: Morgan James Publishing.

Nolfi, K. (1995). *Raw food treatment of cancer*. New York: TEACH Services.

Mikołajczak, N. (2017). Coconut oil in human diet-nutrition value and potential health benefits. *Journal of Education, Health and Sport*, 7 (9), 307-319.

Bassam, N. E. (2015). *Handbook of Bioenergy Crops: A Complete Reference to Species, Development and Applications*. London: Routledge.

Marcin, A. (2017, September 06). Can Coconut Oil Treat Constipation? *Healthline*. Retrieved from https://www.healthline.com/health/coconut-oil-to-treat-constipation.

Allen L. H. (2012). Vitamin B-12. *Advances in nutrition (Bethesda, Md.)*, 3 (1), 54–55.

Sivakumar, B., Nath, N., & Nath, M. C. (1969). Effect of various high protein diets on vitamin B12 status in rats. *The Journal of vitaminology*, 15 (2), 151-154.

Pacholok, S. M., & Stuart, J. J. (2016). *Could it be B12?: What every parent needs to know about vitamin B12 deficiency.* Fresno, California: Quill Driver Books.

Sharabi, A., Cohen, E., Sulkes, J., & Garty, M. (2003). Replacement therapy for vitamin B12 deficiency: comparison between the sublingual and oral route. *British journal of clinical pharmacology, 56* (6), 635–638.

Paul, C., & Brady, D. M. (2017). Comparative bioavailability and utilization of particular forms of B12 supplements with potential to mitigate B12-related genetic polymorphisms. *Integrative Medicine: A Clinician's Journal,* 16 (1), 42.

Sarker, A., Ghosh, A., Sarker, K., Basu, D., & Sen, D. J. (2016). *Halite; The Rock Salt: Enormous Health Benefits.*

Ha S. K. (2014). Dietary salt intake and hypertension. *Electrolyte & blood pressure: E & BP*, 12 (1), 7–18.

Meneton, P., Jeunemaitre, X., de Wardener, H. E., & Macgregor, G. A. (2005). Links between dietary salt intake, renal salt handling, blood pressure, and cardiovascular diseases. *Physiological reviews*, 85 (2), 679-715.

Boero, R., Pignataro, A., & Quarello, F. (2002). Salt intake and kidney disease. *Journal of nephrology*, 15 (3), 225-229.

Sharma, S., & Bhattacharya, A. (2017). Drinking water contamination and treatment techniques. *Applied Water Science, 7* (3), 1043-1067.

Schullehner, J., Hansen, B., Thygesen, M., Pedersen, C. B., & Sigsgaard, T. (2018). Nitrate in drinking water and colorectal cancer risk: A nationwide population-based cohort study.

International journal of cancer, 143 (1), 73-79.

Brewer, G. J. (2019). Avoiding Alzheimer's disease: The important causative role of divalent copper ingestion. *Experimental Biology and Medicine, 244* (2), 114-119.

Singh, I., Sagare, A. P., Coma, M., Perlmutter, D., Gelein, R., Bell, R. D., Deane, R. J., Zhong, E., Parisi, M., Ciszewski, J., Kasper, R. T., & Deane, R. (2013). Low levels of copper disrupt brain amyloid-β homeostasis by altering its production and clearance. *Proceedings of the National Academy of Sciences of the United States of America, 110* (36), 14771–14776.

Brewer, G. J. (2010). Risks of copper and iron toxicity during aging in humans. *Chemical research in toxicology, 23* (2), 319-326.

Gonsioroski, A., Mourikes, V. E., & Flaws, J. A. (2020). Endocrine Disruptors in Water and Their Effects on the Reproductive System. *International journal of molecular sciences, 21* (6), 1929.

George, L. D. (2001). Uses of spring water. In *Springs and Bottled waters of the world* (pp. 105-119). Springer, Berlin, Heidelberg.

Bragg, P. C. (2004). *Water, The Shocking Truth.* United States: Health Science.

Hendry, C. C. (2019). *Ketosis Strips: The Complete User Guide To Using Keto Test Strips To Measure Ketone Levels In Urine And Blood And Getting Into Ketosis Faster.* Amazon Digital Services LLC.

Urbain, P., & Bertz, H. (2016). Monitoring for compliance with a ketogenic diet: what is the best time of day to test for urinary ketosis?. *Nutrition & metabolism*, 13, 77.

Holmer, B. (2019, October 14). Ketones in Urine: All You Need to Know. [Blog post]. Retrieved from https://hvmn.com/blog/ketosis/ketones-in-urine-all-you-need-to-know

Van De Walle, G. (2018, September 18). How to Use Keto Strips to Measure Ketosis. *Healthline.* Retrieved from https://www.healthline.com/nutrition/keto-strips#accuracy

Musa-Veloso, K., Likhodii, S. S., & Cunnane, S. C. (2002). Breath acetone is a reliable indicator of ketosis in adults consuming ketogenic meals. *The American journal of clinical nutrition*, 76 (1), 65-70.

Klocker, A. A., Phelan, H., Twigg, S. M., & Craig, M. E. (2013). Blood β-hydroxybutyrate vs. urine acetoacetate testing for the prevention and management of ketoacidosis in Type 1 diabetes: a systematic review. *Diabetic Medicine*, 30 (7), 818-824.

Wallace, T. M., & Matthews, D. R. (2004). Recent advances in the monitoring and management of diabetic ketoacidosis. *Qjm*, 97 (12), 773-780.

Panoff, L. (2019, June 13). What Is Coconut Meat, and Does It Have Benefits? *Healthline.* Retrieved from https://www.healthline.com/nutrition/coconut-meat#benefits

Fife, B. (2005). *Coconut Cures: Preventing and Treating Common Health Problems with Coconut.* Philippines: Piccadilly Books.

Slavin, J. L. (2008). Position of the American Dietetic Association: health implications of dietary fiber. *Journal of the American Dietetic Association*, *108* (10), 1716-1731.

Coffee Ketosis

Vandenberghe, C., St-Pierre, V., Courchesne-Loyer, A., Hennebelle, M., Castellano, C. A., & Cunnane, S. C. (2016). Caffeine intake increases plasma ketones: an acute metabolic study in humans. *Canadian journal of physiology and pharmacology*, 95 (4), 455-458.

Prasad, S., Tyagi, A. K., & Aggarwal, B. B. (2014). Recent developments in delivery, bioavailability, absorption and metabolism of curcumin: the golden pigment from golden spice. *Cancer research and treatment: official journal of Korean Cancer Association*, *46* (1), 2–18.

Srinivasan, K. (2007). Black pepper and its pungent principle-piperine: a review of diverse physiological effects. *Critical reviews in food science and nutrition*, *47* (8), 735-748.

McCarty, M. F., DiNicolantonio, J. J., & O'Keefe, J. H. (2015). Capsaicin may have important potential for promoting vascular and metabolic health. *Open heart*, *2* (1), e000262.

Macomber, S. (2013). *Our electric emotions: What actually causes mental/emotional illnesses? Is there a way to reverse them?*. Bloomington, Ind.: Xlibris.

Charry, J. M. (2018). *Air Ions: Physical and Biological Aspects.* Boca Raton, FL: CRC Press.

Perez, V., Alexander, D. D., & Bailey, W. H. (2013). Air ions and mood outcomes: a review and meta-analysis. BMC psychiatry, 13, 29.

Russell, W. (1974). *The Universal One*. Swannanoa, Waynesboro, Virginia: University of Science and Philosophy.

Russell, W. (1994). *The Secret of Light*. Swannanoa, Waynesboro, Virginia: University of Science and Philosophy.

Smith, J. J. (2015). *Lose weight without dieting or working out: Discover secrets to a slimmer, sexier, and healthier you*. New York: Atria Books.

Gračanin, A., Bylsma, L. M., & Vingerhoets, A. J. (2014). Is crying a self-soothing behavior?. *Frontiers in psychology*, 5, 502.

Kemp, D., & Daly, P. (2016). *The Ketogenic Kitchen: Low carb. High fat. Extraordinary health*. Dublin: Gill & Macmillan.

Harvey, C., Schofield, G. M., & Williden, M. (2018). The use of nutritional supplements to induce ketosis and reduce symptoms associated with keto-induction: a narrative review. *PeerJ*, 6, e4488.

Mancinelli, K. (2014). *The Ketogenic Diet: A Scientifically Proven Approach to Fast, Healthy Weight Loss*. Berkeley, CA: Ulysses

Spritzler, F., & Scher, B. (2019, May 13). Our comprehensive guide to salt. *Diet Doctor*. Retrieved from https://www.dietdoctor.com/low-carb/salt-guide#on-keto.

McDonald, L., & McDonald, L. (1998). *The ketogenic diet: A complete guide for the dieter and practitioner*. Austin, TX: The Author.

Rodin, J. (1985). Insulin levels, hunger, and food intake: an example of feedback loops in body weight regulation. *Health Psychology*, 4 (1), 1.

Cronometer (2019). *Cronometer: Track Your Nutrition, Fitness, & Health Data, Log your Diet, Exercise, Biometrics and Notes.* Retrieved from https://cronometer.com/

Kalivas, P. W. (2009). The glutamate homeostasis hypothesis of addiction. *Nature reviews neuroscience*, 10 (8), 561.

Cabrera-Mulero, A., Tinahones, A., Bandera, B., Moreno-Indias, I., Macías-González, M., & Tinahones, F. J. (2019). Keto microbiota: a powerful contributor to host disease recovery. *Reviews in Endocrine and Metabolic Disorders*, *20* (4), 415-425.

Mazzoli, R., & Pessione, E. (2016). The Neuro-endocrinological Role of Microbial Glutamate and GABA Signaling. *Frontiers in microbiology*, *7*, 1934.

Abrams, R., Abrams, V. (2019). *Keto Diet For Dummies*. United Kingdom: Wiley.

The Treatment of Obesity. (1979). *United States:* University Park Press.

Pietrzykowski, A. Z., & Treistman, S. N. (2008). The molecular basis of tolerance. *Alcohol research & health: the journal of the National Institute on Alcohol Abuse and Alcoholism*, *31* (4), 298–309.

Sybertz, A. (2020). *The OMAD Diet: Intermittent Fasting with One Meal a Day to Burn Fat and Lose Weight.* United States: Ulysses Press.

Wilkinsen, M. (2019). *The Keto OMAD Diet: How to Combine the Ketogenic Diet with the One Meal A Day Intermittent Fasting Diet to Maximize Your Weight Loss. (n.p.):* INDEPENDENTLY PUBLISHED.

MacDowell, L. (2018). *Vegan Keto.* United States: Victory Belt Publishing.

Fredricks, R. (2012). *Fasting: An Exceptional Human Experience.* United States: AuthorHouse.

Gallagher, E. V, & Willsky-Ciollo, L. (2021*). New Religions: Emerging Faiths and Religious Cultures in the Modern World [2 volumes].* ABC-CLIO.

Kemp, D., & Daly, P. (2016). *The Ketogenic Kitchen: Low carb. High fat. Extraordinary health.* Dublin: Gill & Macmillan.

Saylor, C. P. (2006). *Weight loss, exercise and health research.* New York: Nova Science Publishers.

Moore, J., Rushin, H. (2019). *Keto Clarity Cook book: Your Definitive Guide to Cooking Low-Carb, High-Fat Meals.* United States: Victory Belt Publishing.

Eenfeldt, A. (2021, March 05). How low carb is keto?. *Diet Doctor.* Retrieved from https://www.dietdoctor.com /low-carb/keto/how-low-carb-is-keto

Sunarharum, W. B., Yuwono, S. S., Pangestu, N. B. S. W., & Nadhiroh, H. (2018, March). Physical and sensory quality of Java Arabica green coffee beans. In *IOP Conference Series: Earth and Environmental Science* (Vol. 131, No. 1, p. 012018). IOP Publishing.

Dhillon, K. K., & Gupta, S. (2018). *Biochemistry, Ketogenesis.*

Zuckerman, J. M., & Assimos, D. G. (2009). Hypocitraturia: pathophysiology and medical management. *Reviews in urology, 11* (3), 134–144.

Penniston, K. L., Nakada, S. Y., Holmes, R. P., & Assimos, D. G. (2008). Quantitative assessment of citric acid in lemon juice, lime juice, and commercially-available fruit juice products. *Journal of endourology,* 22 (3), 567–570.

Paoli, A., Bosco, G., Camporesi, E. M., & Mangar, D. (2015). Ketosis, ketogenic diet and food intake control: a complex relationship. *Frontiers in psychology,* 6, 27.

Graham, D. N. (2010). *The 80/10/10 diet: Balancing your health, your weight, and your life one luscious bite at a time.* Key Largo, Fla: FoodnSport Press.

Cousens, G. (2000). *Conscious eating.* Berkeley, Calif: North Atlantic Books.

Cousens, G., & Tree of Life Cafe. (2003). *Rainbow green live-food cuisine.* Berkeley, Calif: North Atlantic Books.

Lee, M. (2017). *Vegan Keto: 70 Healthy & Delicious Low-carb Recipes.* Norway: Pine Peak Publishing.

Nwozo, A. (2019). *The Raw Ketogenic Diet: The Raw Keto Approach to Great Health, Amazing Energy and Permanent Weight Loss Including a 14 day Meal Plan With Net Carbs under 25 g per day!* [Kindle Edition].

Stone, G., Campbell, T. C., & Esselstyn, C. B. (2012). *Forks over knives: The plant-based way to health*. Camberwell, Vic: Penguin Group.

LaBar, D. (2017). *Simple. Natural. Healing: A common sense approach to total health transformation*. New York: Morgan James Publishing.

Nolfi, K. (1995). *Raw food treatment of cancer*. New York: TEACH Services.

Coffee, H. (2018, April 02). 6 Possible Health Benefits of Green Coffee Beans | Raw Coffee Beans | Unroasted Coffee Beans. [Blog]. Retrieved from https://www.haymancoffee.com/blogs/coffee-blog/6-possible-health-benefits-of-green-coffee-beans

Berman, M. (2019, July 8). *Research Shows Green Coffee Beans Does Have Some Proven Benefits.* Healthybutsmart. Retrieved from https://healthybutsmart.com/green-coffee-beans-benefits

Ramalakshmi, K., Kubra, I. R., & Rao, L. J. M. (2007). Physicochemical characteristics of green coffee: Comparison of graded and defective beans. *Journal of food science*, *72* (5), S333-S337.

Clifford, M. N. (1985). Chemical and physical aspects of green coffee and coffee products. In *Coffee* (pp. 305-374). Springer, Boston, MA.

Smith, A. (2002). Effects of caffeine on human behavior. *Food and chemical toxicology*, 40 (9), 1243-1255.

Pray, L., Yaktine, A. L., & Pankevich, D. (2014). Caffeine in food and dietary supplements: examining safety. Workshop summary. In *Caffeine in food and dietary supplements: examining safety. Workshop summary.* National Academies Press.

Rafetto, M., Grumet, T., & French, G. (2004). *Effects of Caffeine and Coffee on Irritable Bowel Syndrome, Crohn's Disease, & Colitis.*

Wolde, T. (2014). Effects of caffeine on health and nutrition: A Review. *Food Science and Quality Management*, 30, 59-65.

Allen L. H. (2012). Vitamin B-12. *Advances in nutrition (Bethesda, Md.)*, 3 (1), 54–55.

Sivakumar, B., Nath, N., & Nath, M. C. (1969). Effect of various high protein diets on vitamin B12 status in rats. *The Journal of vitaminology*, 15 (2), 151-154.

Pacholok, S. M., & Stuart, J. J. (2016). *Could it be B12?: What every parent needs to know about vitamin B12 deficiency.* Fresno, California: Quill Driver Books.

Sharabi, A., Cohen, E., Sulkes, J., & Garty, M. (2003). Replacement therapy for vitamin B12 deficiency: comparison between the sublingual and oral route. *British journal of clinical pharmacology, 56* (6), 635–638.

Paul, C., & Brady, D. M. (2017). Comparative bioavailability and utilization of particular forms of B12 supplements with potential to mitigate B12-related genetic polymorphisms. *Integrative Medicine: A Clinician's Journal,* 16 (1), 42.

Sarker, A., Ghosh, A., Sarker, K., Basu, D., & Sen, D. J. (2016). *Halite; The Rock Salt: Enormous Health Benefits.*

Ha S. K. (2014). Dietary salt intake and hypertension. *Electrolyte & blood pressure: E & BP*, 12 (1), 7–18.

Meneton, P., Jeunemaitre, X., de Wardener, H. E., & Macgregor, G. A. (2005). Links between dietary salt intake, renal salt handling, blood pressure, and cardiovascular diseases. *Physiological reviews*, 85 (2), 679-715.

Boero, R., Pignataro, A., & Quarello, F. (2002). Salt intake and kidney disease. *Journal of nephrology*, 15 (3), 225-229.

Sharma, S., & Bhattacharya, A. (2017). Drinking water contamination and treatment techniques. *Applied Water Science*, 7 (3), 1043-1067.

Schullehner, J., Hansen, B., Thygesen, M., Pedersen, C. B., & Sigsgaard, T. (2018). Nitrate in drinking water and colorectal cancer risk: A nationwide population-based cohort study. *International journal of cancer*, 143 (1), 73-79.

Brewer, G. J. (2019). Avoiding Alzheimer's disease: The important causative role of divalent copper ingestion. *Experimental Biology and Medicine*, 244 (2), 114-119.

Singh, I., Sagare, A. P., Coma, M., Perlmutter, D., Gelein, R., Bell, R. D., Deane, R. J., Zhong, E., Parisi, M., Ciszewski, J., Kasper, R. T., & Deane, R. (2013). Low levels of copper disrupt brain amyloid-β homeostasis by altering its production and clearance. *Proceedings of the National Academy of Sciences of the United States of America, 110* (36), 14771–14776.

Brewer, G. J. (2010). Risks of copper and iron toxicity during aging in humans. *Chemical research in toxicology, 23* (2), 319-326.

Gonsioroski, A., Mourikes, V. E., & Flaws, J. A. (2020). Endocrine Disruptors in Water and Their Effects on the Reproductive System. *International journal of molecular sciences, 21* (6), 1929.

George, L. D. (2001). Uses of spring water. In *Springs and Bottled waters of the world* (pp. 105-119). Springer, Berlin, Heidelberg.

Bragg, P. C. (2004). *Water, The Shocking Truth.* United States: Health Science.

Hendry, C. C. (2019). *Ketosis Strips: The Complete User Guide To Using Keto Test Strips To Measure Ketone Levels In Urine And Blood And Getting Into Ketosis Faster.* Amazon Digital Services LLC.

Urbain, P., & Bertz, H. (2016). Monitoring for compliance with a ketogenic diet: what is the best time of day to test for urinary ketosis?. *Nutrition & metabolism*, 13, 77.

Holmer, B. (2019, October 14). Ketones in Urine: All You Need to Know. [Blog post]. Retrieved from https://hvmn. com/blog/ketosis/ketones-in-urine-all-you-need-to-know

Van De Walle, G. (2018, September 18). How to Use Keto Strips to Measure Ketosis. *Healthline.* Retrieved from https://www.healthline.com/nutrition/keto-strips#accuracy

Musa-Veloso, K., Likhodii, S. S., & Cunnane, S. C. (2002). Breath acetone is a reliable indicator of ketosis in adults consuming ketogenic meals. *The American journal of clinical nutrition*, 76 (1), 65-70.

Klocker, A. A., Phelan, H., Twigg, S. M., & Craig, M. E. (2013). Blood β-hydroxybutyrate vs. urine acetoacetate testing for the prevention and management of ketoacidosis in Type 1 diabetes: a systematic review. *Diabetic Medicine*, 30 (7), 818-824.

Wallace, T. M., & Matthews, D. R. (2004). Recent advances in the monitoring and management of diabetic ketoacidosis. *Qjm*, 97 (12), 773-780.

Bicho, N. C., Lidon, F. C., & Ramalho, J. C. (2013). Quality assessment of Arabica and Robusta green and roasted coffees-A review. *Emirates Journal of Food and Agriculture*, 945-950.

Sunarharum, W. B., Yuwono, S. S., Pangestu, N. B. S. W., & Nadhiroh, H. (2018, March). Physical and sensory quality of Java Arabica green coffee beans. In *IOP Conference Series: Earth and Environmental Science*
(Vol. 131, No. 1, p. 012018). IOP Publishing.

Cacao Ketosis

Vandenberghe, C., St-Pierre, V., Courchesne-Loyer, A., Hennebelle, M., Castellano, C. A., & Cunnane, S. C. (2016). Caffeine intake increases plasma ketones: an acute metabolic study in humans. *Canadian journal of physiology and pharmacology*,95 (4), 455-458.

Norgren, J., Sindi, S., Sandebring-Matton, A., Kåreholt, I., Daniilidou, M., Akenine, U., ... & Kivipelto, M. (2020). Ketosis After Intake of Coconut Oil and Caprylic Acid-With and Without Glucose: A Cross-Over Study in Healthy Older Adults. *Frontiers in nutrition*, 7, 40.

Prasad, S., Tyagi, A. K., & Aggarwal, B. B. (2014). Recent developments in delivery, bioavailability, absorption and metabolism of curcumin: the golden pigment from golden spice. *Cancer research and treatment: official journal of Korean Cancer Association*, *46* (1), 2–18.

Srinivasan, K. (2007). Black pepper and its pungent principle-piperine: a review of diverse physiological effects. *Critical reviews in food science and nutrition*, *47* (8), 735-748.

McCarty, M. F., DiNicolantonio, J. J., & O'Keefe, J. H. (2015). Capsaicin may have important potential for promoting vascular and metabolic health. *Open heart*, *2* (1), e000262.

Clegg, M. E., Golsorkhi, M., & Henry, C. J. (2013). Combined medium-chain triglyceride and chilli feeding increases diet-induced thermogenesis in normal-weight humans. European journal of nutrition, 52 (6), 1579-1585.

Forsyth, W. G. C. (1952). Caffeine in cacao beans. *Nature*, *169* (4288), 33-33.

Charry, J. M. (2018). *Air Ions: Physical and Biological Aspects.* Boca Raton, FL: CRC Press.

Perez, V., Alexander, D. D., & Bailey, W. H. (2013). Air ions and mood outcomes: a review and meta-analysis. BMC psychiatry, 13, 29.

Macomber, S. (2013). *Our electric emotions: What actually causes mental/emotional illnesses? is there a way to reverse them?*. Bloomington, Ind.: Xlibris.

Russell, W. (1974). *The Universal One*. Swannanoa, Waynesboro, Virginia: University of Science and Philosophy.

Russell, W. (1994). *The Secret of Light*. Swannanoa, Waynesboro, Virginia: University of Science and Philosophy.

Smith, J. J. (2015). *Lose weight without dieting or working out: Discover secrets to a slimmer, sexier, and healthier you*. New York: Atria Books.

Chia, M., Dao, J. (2017). The Eight Immortal Healers: Taoist Wisdom for Radiant Health. United States: Inner Traditions/Bear.

Gračanin, A., Bylsma, L. M., & Vingerhoets, A. J. (2014). Is crying a self-soothing behavior?. *Frontiers in psychology*, 5, 502.

Kemp, D., & Daly, P. (2016). *The Ketogenic Kitchen: Low carb. High fat. Extraordinary health*. Dublin: Gill & Macmillan.

Harvey, C., Schofield, G. M., & Williden, M. (2018). The use of nutritional supplements to induce ketosis and reduce symptoms associated with keto-induction: a narrative review. *PeerJ*, 6, e4488.

Mancinelli, K. (2014). *The Ketogenic Diet: A Scientifically Proven Approach to Fast, Healthy Weight Loss*. Berkeley, CA: Ulysses

Spritzler, F., & Scher, B. (2019, May 13). Our comprehensive guide to salt. *Diet Doctor*. Retrieved from https://www.dietdoctor.com/low-carb/salt-guide#on-keto.

McDonald, L., & McDonald, L. (1998). *The ketogenic diet: A complete guide for the dieter and practitioner*. Austin, TX: The Author.

Rodin, J. (1985). Insulin levels, hunger, and food intake: an example of feedback loops in body weight regulation. *Health Psychology*, 4 (1), 1.

Cronometer (2019). *Cronometer: Track Your Nutrition, Fitness, & Health Data, Log your Diet, Exercise, Biometrics and Notes.* Retrieved from https://cronometer.com/

Kalivas, P. W. (2009). The glutamate homeostasis hypothesis of addiction. *Nature reviews neuroscience*, 10 (8), 561.

Cabrera-Mulero, A., Tinahones, A., Bandera, B., Moreno-Indias, I., Macías-González, M., & Tinahones, F. J. (2019). Keto microbiota: a powerful contributor to host disease recovery. *Reviews in Endocrine and Metabolic Disorders*, 20 (4), 415-425.

Mazzoli, R., & Pessione, E. (2016). The Neuro-endocrinological Role of Microbial Glutamate and GABA Signaling. *Frontiers in microbiology*, 7, 1934.

Abrams, R., Abrams, V. (2019). *Keto Diet For Dummies*. United Kingdom: Wiley.

The Treatment of Obesity. (1979). *United States:* University Park Press.

Pietrzykowski, A. Z., & Treistman, S. N. (2008). The molecular basis of tolerance. *Alcohol research & health: the journal of the National Institute on Alcohol Abuse and Alcoholism, 31* (4), 298–309.

Sybertz, A. (2020). *The OMAD Diet: Intermittent Fasting with One Meal a Day to Burn Fat and Lose Weight.* United States: Ulysses Press.

Wilkinsen, M. (2019). *The Keto OMAD Diet: How to Combine the Ketogenic Diet with the One Meal A Day Intermittent Fasting Diet to Maximize Your Weight Loss. (n.p.):* INDEPENDENTLY PUBLISHED.

MacDowell, L. (2018). *Vegan Keto.* United States: Victory Belt Publishing.

Fredricks, R. (2012). *Fasting: An Exceptional Human Experience.* United States: AuthorHouse.

Gallagher, E. V, & Willsky-Ciollo, L. (2021*). New Religions: Emerging Faiths and Religious Cultures in the Modern World [2 volumes].* ABC-CLIO.

Kemp, D., & Daly, P. (2016). *The Ketogenic Kitchen: Low carb. High fat. Extraordinary health.* Dublin: Gill & Macmillan.

Saylor, C. P. (2006). *Weight loss, exercise and healthresearch.* New York: Nova Science Publishers.

Moore, J., Rushin, H. (2019). *Keto Clarity Cook book: Your Definitive Guide to Cooking Low-Carb, High-Fat Meals.* United States: Victory Belt Publishing.

Eenfeldt, A. (2021, March 05). How low carb is keto?. *Diet Doctor.* Retrieved from https://www.dietdoctor.com /low-carb/keto/how-low-carb-is-keto

Dhillon, K. K., & Gupta, S. (2018). *Biochemistry, Ketogenesis.*

Zuckerman, J. M., & Assimos, D. G. (2009). Hypocitraturia: pathophysiology and medical management. *Reviews in urology*, *11* (3), 134–144.

Penniston, K. L., Nakada, S. Y., Holmes, R. P., & Assimos, D. G. (2008). Quantitative assessment of citric acid in lemon juice, lime juice, and commercially-available fruit juice products. *Journal of endourology,* 22 (3), 567–570.

Paoli, A., Bosco, G., Camporesi, E. M., & Mangar, D. (2015). Ketosis, ketogenic diet and food intake control: a complex relationship. *Frontiers in psychology,* 6, 27.

Graham, D. N. (2010). *The 80/10/10 diet: Balancing your health, your weight, and your life one luscious bite at a time.* Key Largo, Fla: FoodnSport Press.

Cousens, G. (2000). *Conscious eating.* Berkeley, Calif: North Atlantic Books.

Cousens, G., & Tree of Life Cafe. (2003). *Rainbow green live-food cuisine*. Berkeley, Calif: North Atlantic Books.

Lee, M. (2017). *Vegan Keto: 70 Healthy & Delicious Low-carb Recipes*. Norway: Pine Peak Publishing.

Nwozo, A. (2019). *The Raw Ketogenic Diet: The Raw Keto Approach to Great Health, Amazing Energy and Permanent Weight Loss Including a 14 day Meal Plan With Net Carbs under 25 g per day!* [Kindle Edition].

Stone, G., Campbell, T. C., & Esselstyn, C. B. (2012). *Forks over knives: The plant-based way to health*. Camberwell, Vic: Penguin Group.

LaBar, D. (2017). *Simple. Natural. Healing: A common sense approach to total health transformation*. New York: Morgan James Publishing.

Nolfi, K. (1995). *Raw food treatment of cancer*. New York: TEACH Services.

de Brito, E. S., García, N. H. P., Gallão, M. I., Cortelazzo, A. L., Fevereiro, P. S., & Braga, M. R. (2001). Structural and chemical changes in cocoa (Theobroma cacao L) during fermentation, drying and roasting. *Journal of the Science of Food and Agriculture, 81* (2), 281-288.

McCulloch, M. (2018, September 10). Cacao vs Cocoa: What's the Difference? *Healthline*. Retrieved from https://www.healthline.com/nutrition/cacao-vs-cocoa

Afoakwa, E. O. (2010). *Chocolate science and technology* (Vol. 687). Oxford: Wiley-Blackwell.

Joel, N., Pius, B., Deborah, A., & Chris, U. (2013). Production and quality evaluation of cocoa products (plain cocoa powder and chocolate). *American journal of food and nutrition, 3* (1), 31-38.

Camu, N., De Winter, T., Addo, S. K., Takrama, J. S., Bernaert, H., & De Vuyst, L. (2008). Fermentation of cocoa beans: influence of microbial activities and polyphenol concentrations on the flavour of chocolate. *Journal of the Science of Food and Agriculture*, *88* (13), 2288-2297.

Kordalis, K. (2019). The Goodness of Raw Chocolate. United Kingdom: Octopus Books.

Wolfe, D., & Shazzie. (2005). *Naked chocolate: The astonishing truth about the world's greatest food*. San Diego: Maul Brothers.

Smith, A. (2002). Effects of caffeine on human behavior. *Food and chemical toxicology*, 40 (9), 1243-1255.

Franco, R., Oñatibia-Astibia, A., & Martínez-Pinilla, E. (2013). Health benefits of methylxanthines in cacao and chocolate. *Nutrients*, 5 (10), 4159–4173.

Pray, L., Yaktine, A. L., & Pankevich, D. (2014). Caffeine in food and dietary supplements: examining safety. Workshop summary. In *Caffeine in food and dietary supplements: examining safety. Workshop summary.* National Academies Press.

Rafetto, M., Grumet, T., & French, G. (2004). *Effects of Caffeine and Coffee on Irritable Bowel Syndrome, Crohn' s Disease, & Colitis.*

Wolde, T. (2014). Effects of caffeine on health and nutrition: A Review. *Food Science and Quality Management*, *30*, 59-65.

JINAP, S., & DIMICK, P. S. (1990). Acidic characteristics of fermented and dried cocoa beans from different countries of origin. *Journal of food science*, 55 (2), 547-550.

Allen L. H. (2012). Vitamin B-12. *Advances in nutrition (Bethesda, Md.)*, 3 (1), 54–55.

Sivakumar, B., Nath, N., & Nath, M. C. (1969). Effect of various high protein diets on vitamin B12 status in rats. *The Journal of vitaminology*, 15 (2), 151-154.

Pacholok, S. M., & Stuart, J. J. (2016). *Could it be B12?: What every parent needs to know about vitamin B12 deficiency*. Fresno, California: Quill Driver Books.

Sharabi, A., Cohen, E., Sulkes, J., & Garty, M. (2003). Replacement therapy for vitamin B12 deficiency: comparison between the sublingual and oral route. *British journal of clinical pharmacology*, *56* (6), 635–638.

Paul, C., & Brady, D. M. (2017). Comparative bioavailability and utilization of particular forms of B12 supplements with potential to mitigate B12-related genetic polymorphisms. *Integrative Medicine: A Clinician's Journal,* 16 (1), 42.

Sarker, A., Ghosh, A., Sarker, K., Basu, D., & Sen, D. J. (2016). *Halite; The Rock Salt: Enormous Health Benefits.*

Ha S. K. (2014). Dietary salt intake and hypertension. *Electrolyte & blood pressure: E & BP*, 12 (1), 7–18.

Meneton, P., Jeunemaitre, X., de Wardener, H. E., & Macgregor, G. A. (2005). Links between dietary salt intake, renal salt handling, blood pressure, and cardiovascular diseases. *Physiological reviews*, 85 (2), 679-715.

Boero, R., Pignataro, A., & Quarello, F. (2002). Salt intake and kidney disease. *Journal of nephrology*, 15 (3), 225-229.

Sharma, S., & Bhattacharya, A. (2017). Drinking water contamination and treatment techniques. *Applied Water Science*, 7 (3), 1043-1067.

Schullehner, J., Hansen, B., Thygesen, M., Pedersen, C. B., & Sigsgaard, T. (2018). Nitrate in drinking water and colorectal cancer risk: A nationwide population-based cohort study. *International journal of cancer*, *143* (1), 73-79.

Brewer, G. J. (2019). Avoiding Alzheimer's disease: The important causative role of divalent copper ingestion. *Experimental Biology and Medicine*, *244* (2), 114-119.

Singh, I., Sagare, A. P., Coma, M., Perlmutter, D., Gelein, R., Bell, R. D., Deane, R. J., Zhong, E., Parisi, M., Ciszewski, J., Kasper, R. T., & Deane, R. (2013). Low levels of copper disrupt brain amyloid-β homeostasis by altering its production and clearance. *Proceedings of the National Academy of Sciences of the United States of America*, *110* (36), 14771–14776.

Brewer, G. J. (2010). Risks of copper and iron toxicity during aging in humans. *Chemical research in toxicology*, *23* (2), 319-326.

Gonsioroski, A., Mourikes, V. E., & Flaws, J. A. (2020). Endocrine Disruptors in Water and Their Effects on the Reproductive System. *International journal of molecular sciences, 21* (6), 1929.

George, L. D. (2001). Uses of spring water. In *Springs and Bottled waters of the world* (pp. 105-119). Springer, Berlin, Heidelberg.

Bragg, P. C. (2004). *Water, The Shocking Truth.* United States: Health Science

Hendry, C. C. (2019). *Ketosis Strips: The Complete User Guide To Using Keto Test Strips To Measure Ketone Levels In Urine And Blood And Getting Into Ketosis Faster.* Amazon Digital Services LLC.

Urbain, P., & Bertz, H. (2016). Monitoring for compliance with a ketogenic diet: what is the best time of day to test for urinary ketosis?. *Nutrition & metabolism*, 13, 77.

Holmer, B. (2019, October 14). Ketones in Urine: All You Need to Know. [Blog post]. Retrieved from https://hvmn .com/blog/ketosis/ketones-in-urine-all-you-need-to-know

Van De Walle, G. (2018, September 18). How to Use Keto Strips to Measure Ketosis. *Healthline.* Retrieved from https://www.healthline.com/nutrition/keto-strips#accuracy

Musa-Veloso, K., Likhodii, S. S., & Cunnane, S. C. (2002). Breath acetone is a reliable indicator of ketosis in adults consuming ketogenic meals. *The American journal of clinical nutrition*, 76 (1), 65-70.

Klocker, A. A., Phelan, H., Twigg, S. M., & Craig, M. E. (2013). Blood β-hydroxybutyrate vs. urine acetoacetate testing for the prevention and management of ketoacidosis in Type 1 diabetes: a systematic review. *Diabetic Medicine*, 30 (7), 818-824.

Wallace, T. M., & Matthews, D. R. (2004). Recent advances in the monitoring and management of diabetic ketoacidosis. *Qjm*, 97 (12), 773-780.

Tea Ketosis

Vandenberghe, C., St-Pierre, V., Courchesne-Loyer, A., Hennebelle, M., Castellano, C. A., & Cunnane, S. C. (2016). Caffeine intake increases plasma ketones: an acute metabolic study in humans. *Canadian journal of physiology and pharmacology*, 95 (4), 455-458.

Prasad, S., Tyagi, A. K., & Aggarwal, B. B. (2014). Recent developments in delivery, bioavailability, absorption and metabolism of curcumin: the golden pigment from golden spice. *Cancer research and treatment: official journal of Korean Cancer Association*, *46* (1), 2–18.

Srinivasan, K. (2007). Black pepper and its pungent principle-piperine: a review of diverse physiological effects. *Critical reviews in food science and nutrition*, *47* (8), 735-748.

McCarty, M. F., DiNicolantonio, J. J., & O'Keefe, J. H. (2015). Capsaicin may have important potential for promoting vascular and metabolic health. *Open heart*, *2* (1), e000262.

Charry, J. M. (2018). *Air Ions: Physical and Biological Aspects.* Boca Raton, FL: CRC Press.

Perez, V., Alexander, D. D., & Bailey, W. H. (2013). Air ions and mood outcomes: a review and meta-analysis. BMC psychiatry, 13, 29.

Macomber, S. (2013). *Our electric emotions: What actually causes mental/emotional illnesses? is there a way to reverse them?*. Bloomington, Ind.: Xlibris.

Russell, W. (1974). *The Universal One.* Swannanoa, Waynesboro, Virginia: University of Science and Philosophy.

Russell, W. (1994). *The Secret of Light*. Swannanoa, Waynesboro, Virginia: University of Science and Philosophy.

Smith, J. J. (2015). *Lose weight without dieting or working out: Discover secrets to a slimmer, sexier, and healthier you*. New York: Atria Books.

Gračanin, A., Bylsma, L. M., & Vingerhoets, A. J. (2014). Is crying a self-soothing behavior?. *Frontiers in psychology*, 5, 502.

Kemp, D., & Daly, P. (2016). *The Ketogenic Kitchen: Low carb. High fat. Extraordinary health*. Dublin: Gill & Macmillan.

Harvey, C., Schofield, G. M., & Williden, M. (2018). The use of nutritional supplements to induce ketosis and reduce symptoms associated with keto-induction: a narrative review. *PeerJ*, 6, e4488.

Mancinelli, K. (2014). *The Ketogenic Diet: A Scientifically Proven Approach to Fast, Healthy Weight Loss*. Berkeley, CA: Ulysses

Spritzler, F., & Scher, B. (2019, May 13). Our comprehensive guide to salt. *Diet Doctor*. Retrieved from https://www.dietdoctor.com/low-carb/salt-guide#on-keto.

McDonald, L., & McDonald, L. (1998). *The ketogenic diet: A complete guide for the dieter and practitioner*. Austin, TX: The Author.

Rodin, J. (1985). Insulin levels, hunger, and food intake: an example of feedback loops in body weight regulation. *Health Psychology*, 4 (1), 1.

Cronometer (2019). *Cronometer: Track Your Nutrition, Fitness, & Health Data, Log your Diet, Exercise, Biometrics and Notes.* Retrieved from https://cronometer.com/

Kalivas, P. W. (2009). The glutamate homeostasis hypothesis of addiction. *Nature reviews neuroscience*, 10 (8), 561.

Cabrera-Mulero, A., Tinahones, A., Bandera, B., Moreno-Indias, I., Macías-González, M., & Tinahones, F. J. (2019). Keto microbiota: a powerful contributor to host disease recovery. *Reviews in Endocrine and Metabolic Disorders*, *20* (4), 415-425.

Mazzoli, R., & Pessione, E. (2016). The Neuro-endocrinological Role of Microbial Glutamate and GABA Signaling. *Frontiers in microbiology*, *7*, 1934.

Abrams, R., Abrams, V. (2019). *Keto Diet For Dummies.* United Kingdom: Wiley.

The Treatment of Obesity. (1979). *United States:* University Park Press.

Pietrzykowski, A. Z., & Treistman, S. N. (2008). The molecular basis of tolerance. *Alcohol research & health: the journal of the National Institute on Alcohol Abuse and Alcoholism*, *31* (4), 298–309.

Sybertz, A. (2020). *The OMAD Diet: Intermittent Fasting with One Meal a Day to Burn Fat and Lose Weight.* United States: Ulysses Press.

Wilkinsen, M. (2019). *The Keto OMAD Diet: How to Combine the Ketogenic Diet with the One Meal A Day Intermittent Fasting Diet to Maximize Your Weight Loss. (n.p.):*

INDEPENDENTLY PUBLISHED.

MacDowell, L. (2018). *Vegan Keto*. United States: Victory Belt Publishing.

Fredricks, R. (2012). *Fasting: An Exceptional Human Experience*. United States: AuthorHouse.

Gallagher, E. V, & Willsky-Ciollo, L. (2021*). New Religions: Emerging Faiths and Religious Cultures in the Modern World [2 volumes]*. ABC-CLIO.

Kemp, D., & Daly, P. (2016). *The Ketogenic Kitchen: Low carb. High fat. Extraordinary health*. Dublin: Gill & Macmillan.

Saylor, C. P. (2006). *Weight loss, exercise and health research*. New York: Nova Science Publishers.

Moore, J., Rushin, H. (2019). *Keto Clarity Cookbook: Your Definitive Guide to Cooking Low-Carb, High-Fat Meals*. United States: Victory Belt Publishing.

Eenfeldt, A. (2021, March 05). How low carb is keto?. *Diet Doctor*. Retrieved from https://www.dietdoctor.com/low-carb/keto/how-low-carb-is-keto

Cloughley, J. B. (1982). Factors influencing the caffeine content of black tea: Part 1 - The effect of field variables. *Food Chemistry, 9* (4), 269-276.

Dhillon, K. K., & Gupta, S. (2018). *Biochemistry, Ketogenesis.*

Zuckerman, J. M., & Assimos, D. G. (2009). Hypocitraturia: pathophysiology and medical management. *Reviews in urology, 11* (3), 134–144.

Penniston, K. L., Nakada, S. Y., Holmes, R. P., & Assimos, D. G. (2008). Quantitative assessment of citric acid in lemon juice, lime juice, and commercially-available fruit juice products. *Journal of endourology,* 22 (3), 567–570.

Paoli, A., Bosco, G., Camporesi, E. M., & Mangar, D. (2015). Ketosis, ketogenic diet and food intake control: a complex relationship. *Frontiers in psychology,* 6, 27.

Graham, D. N. (2010). *The 80/10/10 diet: Balancing your health, your weight, and your life one luscious bite at a time.* Key Largo, Fla: FoodnSport Press.

Cousens, G. (2000). *Conscious eating.* Berkeley, Calif: North Atlantic Books.

Cousens, G., & Tree of Life Cafe. (2003). *Rainbow green live-food cuisine*. Berkeley, Calif: North Atlantic Books.

Lee, M. (2017). *Vegan Keto: 70 Healthy & Delicious Low-carb Recipes*. Norway: Pine Peak Publishing.

Nwozo, A. (2019). *The Raw Ketogenic Diet: The Raw Keto Approach to Great Health, Amazing Energy and Permanent Weight Loss Including a 14 day Meal Plan With Net Carbs under 25 g per day!* [Kindle Edition].

Stone, G., Campbell, T. C., & Esselstyn, C. B. (2012). *Forks over knives: The plant-based way to health*. Camberwell, Vic: Penguin Group.

LaBar, D. (2017). *Simple. Natural. Healing: A common sense approach to total health transformation*. New York: Morgan James Publishing.

Nolfi, K. (1995). *Raw food treatment of cancer*. New York: TEACH Services.

Smith, A. (2002). Effects of caffeine on human behavior. *Food and chemical toxicology*, 40 (9), 1243-1255.

Pray, L., Yaktine, A. L., & Pankevich, D. (2014). Caffeine in food and dietary supplements: examining safety. Workshop summary. In *Caffeine in food and dietary supplements: examining safety. Workshop summary*. National Academies Press.

Rafetto, M., Grumet, T., & French, G. (2004). *Effects of Caffeine and Coffee on Irritable Bowel Syndrome, Crohn's Disease, & Colitis*.

Wolde, T. (2014). Effects of caffeine on health and nutrition: A Review. *Food Science and Quality Management*, 30, 59-65.

Kohlmeier, L. (1997). Has the tea been ruined?. *British Journal of Nutrition*, 78 (1), 1-3.

Allen L. H. (2012). Vitamin B-12. *Advances in nutrition (Bethesda, Md.)*, 3 (1), 54–55.

Sivakumar, B., Nath, N., & Nath, M. C. (1969). Effect of various high protein diets on vitamin B12 status in rats. *The Journal of vitaminology*, 15 (2), 151-154.

Pacholok, S. M., & Stuart, J. J. (2016). *Could it be B12?: What every parent needs to know about vitamin B12 deficiency*. Fresno, California: Quill Driver Books.

Sharabi, A., Cohen, E., Sulkes, J., & Garty, M. (2003). Replacement therapy for vitamin B12 deficiency: comparison between the sublingual and oral route. *British journal of clinical pharmacology*, *56* (6), 635–638.

Paul, C., & Brady, D. M. (2017). Comparative bioavailability and utilization of particular forms of B12 supplements with potential to mitigate B12-related genetic polymorphisms. *Integrative Medicine: A Clinician's Journal,* 16 (1), 42.

Sarker, A., Ghosh, A., Sarker, K., Basu, D., & Sen, D. J. (2016). *Halite; The Rock Salt: Enormous Health Benefits.*

Ha S. K. (2014). Dietary salt intake and hypertension. *Electrolyte & blood pressure: E & BP*, 12 (1), 7–18.

Meneton, P., Jeunemaitre, X., de Wardener, H. E., & Macgregor, G. A. (2005). Links between dietary salt intake, renal salt handling, blood pressure, and cardiovascular diseases. *Physiological reviews*, 85 (2), 679-715.

Boero, R., Pignataro, A., & Quarello, F. (2002). Salt intake and kidney disease. *Journal of nephrology*, 15 (3), 225-229.

Sharma, S., & Bhattacharya, A. (2017). Drinking water contamination and treatment techniques. *Applied Water Science*, *7* (3), 1043-1067.

Schullehner, J., Hansen, B., Thygesen, M., Pedersen, C. B., & Sigsgaard, T. (2018). Nitrate in drinking water and colorectal cancer risk: A nationwide population-based cohort study. *International journal of cancer*, *143* (1), 73-79.

Brewer, G. J. (2019). Avoiding Alzheimer's disease: The important causative role of divalent copper ingestion. *Experimental Biology and Medicine, 244* (2), 114-119.

Singh, I., Sagare, A. P., Coma, M., Perlmutter, D., Gelein, R., Bell, R. D., Deane, R. J., Zhong, E., Parisi, M., Ciszewski, J., Kasper, R. T., & Deane, R. (2013). Low levels of copper disrupt brain amyloid-β homeostasis by altering its production and clearance. *Proceedings of the National Academy of Sciences of the United States of America, 110* (36), 14771–14776.

Brewer, G. J. (2010). Risks of copper and iron toxicity during aging in humans. *Chemical research in toxicology, 23* (2), 319-326.

Gonsioroski, A., Mourikes, V. E., & Flaws, J. A. (2020). Endocrine Disruptors in Water and Their Effects on the Reproductive System. *International journal of molecular sciences, 21* (6), 1929.

George, L. D. (2001). Uses of spring water. In *Springs and Bottled waters of the world* (pp. 105-119). Springer, Berlin, Heidelberg.

Bragg, P. C. (2004). *Water, The Shocking Truth.* United States: Health Science.

Hendry, C. C. (2019). *Ketosis Strips: The Complete User Guide To Using Keto Test Strips To Measure Ketone Levels In Urine And Blood And Getting Into Ketosis Faster.* Amazon Digital Services LLC.

Urbain, P., & Bertz, H. (2016). Monitoring for compliance with a ketogenic diet: what is the best time of day to test for urinary ketosis?. *Nutrition & metabolism, 13,* 77.

Holmer, B. (2019, October 14). Ketones in Urine: All You Need to Know. [Blog post]. Retrieved from https://hvmn.com /blog/ketosis/ketones-in-urine-all-you-need-to-know

Van De Walle, G. (2018, September 18). How to Use Keto Strips to Measure Ketosis. *Healthline.* Retrieved from https://www.healthline.com/nutrition/keto-strips #accuracy

Musa-Veloso, K., Likhodii, S. S., & Cunnane, S. C. (2002). Breath acetone is a reliable indicator of ketosis in adults consuming ketogenic meals. *The American journal of clinical nutrition*, 76 (1), 65-70.

Klocker, A. A., Phelan, H., Twigg, S. M., & Craig, M. E. (2013). Blood β-hydroxybutyrate vs. urine acetoacetate testing for the prevention and management of ketoacidosis in Type 1 diabetes: a systematic review. *Diabetic Medicine*, 30 (7), 818-824.

Wallace, T. M., & Matthews, D. R. (2004). Recent advances in the monitoring and management of diabetic ketoacidosis. *Qjm*, 97 (12), 773-780.

Matcha Ketosis

Vandenberghe, C., St-Pierre, V., Courchesne-Loyer, A., Hennebelle, M., Castellano, C. A., & Cunnane, S. C. (2016). Caffeine intake increases plasma ketones: an acute metabolic study in humans. *Canadian journal of physiology and pharmacology*, 95 (4), 455-458.

Prasad, S., Tyagi, A. K., & Aggarwal, B. B. (2014). Recent developments in delivery, bioavailability, absorption and metabolism of curcumin: the golden pigment from golden spice. *Cancer research and treatment: official journal of Korean Cancer Association*, *46* (1), 2–18.

Srinivasan, K. (2007). Black pepper and its pungent principle-piperine: a review of diverse physiological effects. *Critical reviews in food science and nutrition*, *47* (8), 735-748.

McCarty, M. F., DiNicolantonio, J. J., & O'Keefe, J. H. (2015). Capsaicin may have important potential for promoting vascular and metabolic health. *Open heart*, *2* (1), e000262.

Charry, J. M. (2018). *Air Ions: Physical and Biological Aspects.* Boca Raton, FL: CRC Press.

Perez, V., Alexander, D. D., & Bailey, W. H. (2013). Air ions and mood outcomes: a review and meta-analysis. BMC psychiatry, 13, 29.

Macomber, S. (2013). *Our electric emotions: What actually causes mental/emotional illnesses? is there a way to reverse them?.* Bloomington, Ind.: Xlibris.

Russell, W. (1974). *The Universal One.* Swannanoa, Waynesboro, Virginia: University of Science and Philosophy.

Russell, W. (1994). *The Secret of Light.* Swannanoa, Waynesboro, Virginia: University of Science and Philosophy.

Smith, J. J. (2015). *Lose weight without dieting or working out: Discover secrets to a slimmer, sexier, and healthier you.* New York: Atria Books.

Gračanin, A., Bylsma, L. M., & Vingerhoets, A. J. (2014). Is crying a self-soothing behavior?. *Frontiers in psychology*, 5, 502.

Kemp, D., & Daly, P. (2016). *The Ketogenic Kitchen: Low carb. High fat. Extraordinary health*. Dublin: Gill & Macmillan.

Harvey, C., Schofield, G. M., & Williden, M. (2018). The use of nutritional supplements to induce ketosis and reduce symptoms associated with keto-induction: a narrative review. *PeerJ*, 6, e4488.

Mancinelli, K. (2014). *The Ketogenic Diet: A Scientifically Proven Approach to Fast, Healthy Weight Loss*. Berkeley, CA: Ulysses

Spritzler, F., & Scher, B. (2019, May 13). Our comprehensive guide to salt. *Diet Doctor*. Retrieved from https://www.dietdoctor.com/low-carb/salt-guide#on-keto.

McDonald, L., & McDonald, L. (1998). *The ketogenic diet: A complete guide for the dieter and practitioner*. Austin, TX: The Author.

Rodin, J. (1985). Insulin levels, hunger, and food intake: an example of feedback loops in body weight regulation. *Health Psychology*, 4 (1), 1.

Cronometer (2019). *Cronometer: Track Your Nutrition, Fitness, & Health Data, Log your Diet, Exercise, Biometrics and Notes.* Retrieved from https://cronometer.com/

Kalivas, P. W. (2009). The glutamate homeostasis hypothesis of addiction. *Nature reviews neuroscience*, 10 (8), 561.

Cabrera-Mulero, A., Tinahones, A., Bandera, B., Moreno-Indias, I., Macías-González, M., & Tinahones, F. J. (2019). Keto microbiota: a powerful contributor to host disease recovery. *Reviews in Endocrine and Metabolic Disorders*,

20 (4), 415-425.

Mazzoli, R., & Pessione, E. (2016). The Neuro-endocrinological Role of Microbial Glutamate and GABA Signaling. *Frontiers in microbiology*, *7*, 1934.

Abrams, R., Abrams, V. (2019). *Keto Diet For Dummies.* United Kingdom: Wiley.

The Treatment of Obesity. (1979). *United States:* University Park Press.

Pietrzykowski, A. Z., & Treistman, S. N. (2008). The molecular basis of tolerance. *Alcohol research & health: the journal of the National Institute on Alcohol Abuse and Alcoholism*, *31* (4), 298–309.

Sybertz, A. (2020). *The OMAD Diet: Intermittent Fasting with One Meal a Day to Burn Fat and Lose Weight.* United States: Ulysses Press.

Wilkinsen, M. (2019). *The Keto OMAD Diet: How to Combine the Ketogenic Diet with the One Meal A Day Intermittent Fasting Diet to Maximize Your Weight Loss. (n.p.):* INDEPENDENTLY PUBLISHED.

MacDowell, L. (2018). *Vegan Keto.* United States: Victory Belt Publishing.

Fredricks, R. (2012). *Fasting: An Exceptional Human Experience.* United States: AuthorHouse.

Gallagher, E. V, & Willsky-Ciollo, L. (2021*). New Religions: Emerging Faiths and Religious Cultures in the Modern World [2 volumes].* ABC-CLIO.

Saylor, C. P. (2006). *Weight loss, exercise and health research*. New York: Nova Science Publishers.

Moore, J., Rushin, H. (2019). *Keto Clarity Cook book: Your Definitive Guide to Cooking Low-Carb, High-Fat Meals*. United States: Victory Belt Publishing.

Eenfeldt, A. (2021, March 05). How low carb is keto?. *Diet Doctor*. Retrieved from https://www.dietdoctor.com/low-carb/keto/how-low-carb-is-keto

CAI, J. X., REN, J., LI, C. F., WANG, W. T., WEI, X. L., & WANG, Y. F. (2015). Effect of different fixing methods on the quality of selenium-enriched matcha. *Science and Technology of Food Industry*, *2015* (14), 41.

Komes, D., Horžić, D., Belščak, A., Ganić, K. K., & Vulić, I. (2010). Green tea preparation and its influence on the content of bioactive compounds. Food research international, 43 (1), 167-176.

Dhillon, K. K., & Gupta, S. (2018). *Biochemistry, Ketogenesis.*

Zuckerman, J. M., & Assimos, D. G. (2009). Hypocitraturia: pathophysiology and medical management. *Reviews in urology*, *11* (3), 134–144.

Penniston, K. L., Nakada, S. Y., Holmes, R. P., & Assimos, D. G. (2008). Quantitative assessment of citric acid in lemon juice, lime juice, and commercially-available fruit juice products. *Journal of endourology,* 22 (3), 567–570.

Paoli, A., Bosco, G., Camporesi, E. M., & Mangar, D. (2015). Ketosis, ketogenic diet and food intake control: a complex relationship. *Frontiers in psychology,* 6, 27.

Graham, D. N. (2010). *The 80/10/10 diet: Balancing your health, your weight, and your life one luscious bite at a time.* Key Largo, Fla: FoodnSport Press.

Cousens, G. (2000). *Conscious eating.* Berkeley, Calif: North Atlantic Books.

Cousens, G., & Tree of Life Cafe. (2003). *Rainbow green live-food cuisine*. Berkeley, Calif: North Atlantic Books.

Lee, M. (2017). *Vegan Keto: 70 Healthy & Delicious Low-carb Recipes*. Norway: Pine Peak Publishing.

Nwozo, A. (2019). *The Raw Ketogenic Diet: The Raw Keto Approach to Great Health, Amazing Energy and Permanent Weight Loss Including a 14 day Meal Plan With Net Carbs under 25 g per day!* [Kindle Edition].

Stone, G., Campbell, T. C., & Esselstyn, C. B. (2012). *Forks over knives: The plant-based way to health*. Camberwell, Vic: Penguin Group.

LaBar, D. (2017). *Simple. Natural. Healing: A common sense approach to total health transformation*. New York: Morgan James Publishing.

Nolfi, K. (1995). *Raw food treatment of cancer*. New York: TEACH Services.

Smith, A. (2002). Effects of caffeine on human behavior. *Food and chemical toxicology,* 40 (9), 1243-1255.

Pray, L., Yaktine, A. L., & Pankevich, D. (2014). Caffeine in food and dietary supplements: examining safety. Workshop summary. In *Caffeine in food and dietary supplements: examining safety. Workshop summary.* National Academies Press.

Rafetto, M., Grumet, T., & French, G. (2004). *Effects of Caffeine and Coffee on Irritable Bowel Syndrome, Crohn' s Disease, & Colitis.*

Wolde, T. (2014). Effects of caffeine on health and nutrition: A Review. *Food Science and Quality Management*, 30, 59-65.

Kohlmeier, L. (1997). Has the tea been ruined?. *British Journal of Nutrition*, 78 (1), 1-3.

Brown, H. (2019, January 18). *16 Evidence-Based Health Benefits of Matcha Tea.* Well-Being Secrets. Retrieved from https://www.well-beingsecrets.com/matcha-tea-benefits/

Weiss, D. J., & Anderton, C. R. (2003). Determination of catechins in matcha green tea by micellar electrokinetic chromatography. *Journal of Chromatography A*, *1011* (1-2), 173-180.

Allen L. H. (2012). Vitamin B-12. *Advances in nutrition (Bethesda, Md.)*, 3 (1), 54–55.

Sivakumar, B., Nath, N., & Nath, M. C. (1969). Effect of various high protein diets on vitamin B12 status in rats. *The Journal of vitaminology*, 15 (2), 151-154.

Pacholok, S. M., & Stuart, J. J. (2016). *Could it be B12?: What every parent needs to know about vitamin B12 deficiency.* Fresno, California: Quill Driver Books.

Sharabi, A., Cohen, E., Sulkes, J., & Garty, M. (2003). Replacement therapy for vitamin B12 deficiency: comparison between the sublingual and oral route. *British journal of clinical pharmacology*, *56* (6), 635–638.

Paul, C., & Brady, D. M. (2017). Comparative bioavailability and utilization of particular forms of B12 supplements with potential to mitigate B12-related genetic polymorphisms. *Integrative Medicine: A Clinician's Journal,* 16 (1), 42.

Sarker, A., Ghosh, A., Sarker, K., Basu, D., & Sen, D. J. (2016). *Halite; The Rock Salt: Enormous Health Benefits.*

Ha S. K. (2014). Dietary salt intake and hypertension. *Electrolyte & blood pressure: E & BP*, 12 (1), 7–18.

Meneton, P., Jeunemaitre, X., de Wardener, H. E., & Macgregor, G. A. (2005). Links between dietary salt intake, renal salt handling, blood pressure, and cardiovascular diseases. *Physiological reviews*, 85 (2), 679-715.

Boero, R., Pignataro, A., & Quarello, F. (2002). Salt intake and kidney disease. *Journal of nephrology*, 15 (3), 225-229.

Sharma, S., & Bhattacharya, A. (2017). Drinking water contamination and treatment techniques. *Applied Water Science*, *7* (3), 1043-1067.

Schullehner, J., Hansen, B., Thygesen, M., Pedersen, C. B., & Sigsgaard, T. (2018). Nitrate in drinking water and colorectal cancer risk: A nationwide population-based cohort study. *International journal of cancer*, *143* (1), 73-79.

Brewer, G. J. (2019). Avoiding Alzheimer's disease: The important causative role of divalent copper ingestion. *Experimental Biology and Medicine*, *244* (2), 114-119.

Singh, I., Sagare, A. P., Coma, M., Perlmutter, D., Gelein, R., Bell, R. D., Deane, R. J., Zhong, E., Parisi, M., Ciszewski, J., Kasper, R. T., & Deane, R. (2013). Low levels of copper disrupt brain amyloid-β homeostasis by altering its production and clearance. *Proceedings of the National Academy of Sciences of the United States of America*, *110* (36), 14771–14776.

Brewer, G. J. (2010). Risks of copper and iron toxicity during aging in humans. *Chemical research in toxicology*, *23* (2), 319-326.

Gonsioroski, A., Mourikes, V. E., & Flaws, J. A. (2020). Endocrine Disruptors in Water and Their Effects on the Reproductive System. *International journal of molecular sciences, 21* (6), 1929.

George, L. D. (2001). Uses of spring water. In *Springs and Bottled waters of the world* (pp. 105-119). Springer, Berlin, Heidelberg.

Bragg, P. C. (2004). *Water, The Shocking Truth.* United States: Health Science.

Hendry, C. C. (2019). *Ketosis Strips: The Complete User Guide To Using Keto Test Strips To Measure Ketone Levels In Urine And Blood And Getting Into Ketosis Faster.* Amazon Digital Services LLC.

Urbain, P., & Bertz, H. (2016). Monitoring for compliance with a ketogenic diet: what is the best time of day to test for urinary ketosis?. *Nutrition & metabolism*, 13, 77.

Holmer, B. (2019, October 14). Ketones in Urine: All You Need to Know. [Blog post]. Retrieved from https://hvmn.com/blog/ketosis/ketones-in-urine-all-you-need-to-know

Van De Walle, G. (2018, September 18). How to Use Keto Strips to Measure Ketosis. *Healthline.* Retrieved from https://www.healthline.com/nutrition/keto-strips#accuracy

Musa-Veloso, K., Likhodii, S. S., & Cunnane, S. C. (2002). Breath acetone is a reliable indicator of ketosis in adults consuming ketogenic meals. *The American journal of clinical nutrition*, 76 (1), 65-70.

Klocker, A. A., Phelan, H., Twigg, S. M., & Craig, M. E. (2013). Blood β-hydroxybutyrate vs. urine acetoacetate testing for the prevention and management of ketoacidosis in Type 1 diabetes: a systematic review. *Diabetic Medicine*, 30 (7), 818-824.

Wallace, T. M., & Matthews, D. R. (2004). Recent advances in the monitoring and management of diabetic ketoacidosis. *Qjm*, 97 (12), 773-780.

Made in the USA
Columbia, SC
27 June 2023